T0299647

# Hope and Healing after Stillbirth and New Baby Loss

PROFESSOR KEVIN GOURNAY
&
DR BRENDA ASHCROFT

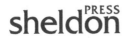

First published in Great Britain in 2019 by Sheldon Press,
an imprint of John Murray Learning.
An Hachette UK company.

This edition first published by Sheldon Press in 2024
An imprint of John Murray Press

1

A CIP catalogue record for this title is available from the British Library

Trade Paperback ISBN 978 1 399 81646 5
ebook ISBN 978 1 399 81650 2

Typeset by KnowledgeWorks Global Ltd.

Printed and bound in Great Britain by Clays Ltd, Elcograf S.p.A.

John Murray Press policy is to use papers that are natural, renewable and
recyclable products and made from wood grown in sustainable forests.
The logging and manufacturing processes are expected to conform to
the environmental regulations of the country of origin.

John Murray Press
Carmelite House
50 Victoria Embankment
London EC4Y 0DZ

www.sheldonpress.co.uk

John Murray Press, part of Hodder & Stoughton Limited
An Hachette UK company

*In loving memory of Georgina – never forgotten – and all other lost babies, too many to mention.*

# Contents

# Foreword

When I was elected as the Member of Parliament for Lewisham Deptford in 2015, I had no idea that I would end up sharing my most painful memories in the House of Commons.

In the days leading up to the 2016 Baby Loss Awareness Week debate I battled with the idea of talking about Veronica, the daughter I had lost 23 years previously at just five days old. Only my very closest friends and family knew about her and I still find her birth and death difficult to talk about.

But when the day came, I knew I had to do it. It was the first ever full Commons debate on baby loss and I realized how much it would mean to the thousands of parents who have been through the same traumatic experience. In the days that followed I received hundreds of emails from people wanting to share their experiences.

In recent decades, stillbirth and neonatal death rates have steadily fallen in the UK. However, when the data is broken down by region, ethnicity and deprivation, significant and persistent inequalities are exposed. The most recent data – published since the first edition of this book came out – also indicates that progress is slowing (or even reversing in some areas) and that experiences of care are deteriorating.

The ultimate goal is to prevent neonatal deaths from happening in the first place. However, our current priority must be to ensure that appropriate support is available to the parents who are experiencing loss in the here and now, as well as to the healthcare professionals who work with them.

I applaud everyone who is working to break the silence around stillbirth and neonatal death. No parent expects to find themselves in such a devastating situation and that is why books like this one are so important.

I am delighted to introduce the second edition and I hope it will help many more parents navigate their way through a complex and traumatic time.

Vicky Foxcroft, MP

# About this book

One woman said six months after the experience of a stillbirth:

> This tragedy has affected my whole life ... my relationships,
> my job, and just the way I look at life now ... I now have so
> many emotions, they are still in turmoil; anxiety, depression,
> anger, feelings that I want to end things here and now and, in
> the quiet of the early morning, guilt and recrimination about
> what I don't know ...

## A note about the focus of this book

After much thought, the authors decided that the focus of this
book should be on the early loss of a baby. This includes babies
who died in the womb and were then stillborn, and babies who
died in the early days and weeks of life.

## Our readership

When we set out to write this book our intended readership was
the large number of those parents directly affected by this loss.
However, on completing the writing we came to the realization
that there are many health professionals whose knowledge of
this topic is superficial to say the least. Even of those in the 'front
line' who come across women and their partners who have been
so affected, many have little idea of the long-term impact and
importantly have little, or no, knowledge of what might be done
to alleviate the suffering and emotional pain that may continue,
unremittingly, for months or even years after the original event.
We therefore hope that the readership of this book might extend
beyond affected individuals.

## A note of caution

Although this book is primarily intended to provide information and to assist with coping and recovery from the tragic events that are the subject of this book, we realize that parents and others may well find reading some parts of this book difficult and, at times, possibly distressing. We know from our own experience that hearing the stories of others is at once upsetting but also of comfort in knowing that one is not alone. Some parts of this book may set off thoughts and feelings that cause distress, discomfort, anxiety or other emotions. Although we hope that none of the above reactions occurs, we know that overcoming the traumatic impact of losing a child is inevitably a painful process.

Although some people prefer to read a book from cover to cover or in large chunks, you might want to limit yourself to reading short sections at a time and then putting the book down and going on to other more pleasurable distractions. This is also a book that you can dip into, so when you look at the Contents or the Index, you might find a section that particularly applies to you – for example, coping with a particular feeling. By all means dip in and out, but try, over time, to finish the entire book. Some of you may also find it helpful to make notes as you go along.

A final note of caution: should reading this book produce any overwhelming distress that does not readily subside once you have put down the book, you should, before continuing, discuss your reactions with your GP or, if you are undergoing treatment, with your medical specialist or therapist.

## A note about same-sex couples

The advent of in vitro fertilization (IVF) has served to produce another dimension to the topic. Throughout the book we have used the word 'partners' rather than fathers so as to acknowledge the fact that stillbirth and early death affects same-sex couples as well. One of the authors has seen the effect of stillbirth on a woman and her female partner and therefore, through this experience, has come to the clear view that same-sex couples are as vulnerable to suffering the same consequences as male and female couples. As far as same-sex male couples who have experienced the loss of a baby, carried through pregnancy by a surrogate, one can only speculate that there will be consequent distress for all those involved. The authors simply wish to say that they acknowledge these developments and to confirm their commitment to treating all those affected with the same respect and commitment to do whatever they can for those who have suffered such a tragedy.

## The case histories within this book

Based on the experience of writing books on coping with various topics and hearing the response of readers, we have used case studies to illustrate the nature of the issue and to show that what one can do for oneself can result in beneficial outcomes. We have also included case histories to illustrate a number of important points. All the descriptions come from our own clinical experiences, gathered over many years. However, we have protected the anonymity of particular individuals not only by changing names, but also by a process of interchanging parts of the history (that is, events and signs and symptoms). However, everything set out in the histories is true.

## The role of Sands

Throughout, this book we have mentioned the Stillbirth and Neonatal Death Society (Sands). Both authors have considerable experience of Sands. We are of the opinion that this organization has made a great contribution not only to parents and sometimes their families, but also to the professionals involved in this area. Our emphasis on Sands does not in any way diminish the efforts of other similar organizations. At the end of this book there is a section that provides contact details for other organizations that provide invaluable support and information.

Sands was founded in 1978 by a small group of bereaved parents. Since then it has become the UK's leading organization providing help and support for families bereaved by stillbirth, neonatal death and miscarriage. Every year Sands helps thousands of families who have been affected by the loss of a baby, by focusing on three key areas. These are providing support for anyone affected by the death of a baby, working in partnership with professionals to try to ensure that bereaved parents and families receive the best possible care, and finally promoting and funding research to help reduce the loss of babies. Many people who have benefited from their support have later become ardent fundraisers for the charity, which relies on public donations to deliver its wide range of services.

Sands has a UK network of local support groups, which are run by dedicated volunteers who have undergone training in befriending and providing peer support to anybody affected by the loss of a baby. The volunteers themselves have very often experienced this type of loss, enabling them to personally relate to other bereaved families. The local groups offer a wide range of support services, including a helpline for parents, families, carers and health professionals. There is also an online forum and message board enabling bereaved families to connect with others, and a website listing a wide range of books, leaflets and other resources. In addition to this they provide every family with a Family Support Pack and an Always Loved Never Forgotten memory box. These will be described later in more detail. Information and support for anyone affected by the death of a baby can contact the Sands Helpline on a free number: 0808 164332, or via email at: <helpline@uk-sands.org>.

# Introduction

This book is the result of the collective experience of two authors who between them have more than six decades of experience of dealing with women and their partners who have experienced the loss of a baby, either by stillbirth or from the death of a baby shortly after birth. Why, then, this book at this particular time? Both of us have been deeply touched by our experiences as professionals of seeing the devastating effects of such loss and, at the same time, realizing that the effects of this tragic loss may be long-lasting and – not to overdramatize it – in some cases life-changing.

We have both been aware that many affected individuals are simply left to their own devices, and that professional help, when available, is often inadequate to meet their needs. While we applaud the efforts of organizations such as Sands to provide help, support and advice, and indeed the efforts of a small number of authors who have written excellent books on the topic, we came to the view that what was needed was a book that provided information, but also could provide advice on developing ways of coping. The recent and very welcome efforts of the UK Parliament have raised awareness of the breadth and depth of the problems resulting from stillbirth and perinatal death (the latter relating to the time immediately before, during and after birth), and this has also inspired us to publish a book at this particular time, as increasing awareness of the problem is just the first step in what is needed.

We realize that, if you have suffered the loss of a baby, reading this book may be a very difficult. As we have noted above, we have laid out the content in such a way that topics can be chosen and read as stand-alone items. For example, you might find that you want to read about the professional or voluntary sector resources available to help you. The authors bring different perspectives in their approach to this book, but both agree that the loss of a baby, either before or shortly after birth, is a tragic and heart-breaking event and one that will never be forgotten, even after many years.

As a midwife, Brenda Ashcroft knows that the midwives involved in providing care for the mother at this time will also feel their own sense of sorrow as their role is aimed at bringing live babies into the world. From Brenda's own experience as a midwife, she can say that providing care to the mother who has lost her baby is heart-rending and emotionally demanding. Nonetheless, it is a very important part of a midwife's role because a mother and her family will never forget the events surrounding their loss and the midwives' care.

Kevin Gournay has been fortunate enough to be present at the birth of his own children and, in his student days, was present at the caesarean births of babies to mothers whom he did not know. These occasions provided joyful memories that he will never forget. By contrast, his experience as a psychologist of women who have suffered the tragedy of the death of a baby comes from meeting these women (and sometimes their husbands or partners) months or, in some cases, years after. In listening to women telling their own, unique story Kevin has realized that these women are describing events that will never be adequately expressed in words and, in accord with Brenda's experience, such a loss will never be forgotten.

We know that this book may be the most difficult read of your life. However, we have a sincere hope that this might provide the missing 'something' that will prove to be the difference between coping and not coping.

# Part 1
# CONSEQUENCES

# 1

# Consequences of stillbirth and early death

We began this book quoting the experience of one woman who said, six months after she had given birth to a stillborn child:

> This tragedy has affected my whole life ... my relationships, my job, and just the way I look at life now ... I now have so many emotions, they are still in turmoil; anxiety, depression, anger, feelings that I want to end things here and now and, in the quiet of the early morning, guilt and recrimination about what I don't know ...

Although many of the emotions that arise following this heart-breaking loss are shared by the vast majority of women and their partners, we also know, at the same time, that each person has a unique story. Even when women and their partners sometimes sit in the same room at a support group, with someone saying 'I know how you feel', this statement is only partially correct. In this section we will set out what is known about the consequences of such loss. In Part 3 of this book, we provide advice and information on dealing with some commonly encountered problems.

## What does research tell us?

One of the most comprehensive accounts of stillbirth and early baby loss is provided in a review published in 2016 by an international research group (*The Lancet*, 2016) This review described the economic, psychological and social consequences of stillbirth and early death. The group of researchers came from Australia, Norway, Switzerland and the UK, and they collected a wide range of information concerning the psychological and social effects by examining the results of a number of research studies in different countries. The authors also examined the financial costs and, particularly, the effect of stillbirth on the employment of affected parents.

With regard to the emotional and psychological consequences of stillbirth on parents, it was reported that 77 per cent of parents were affected. Of considerable concern, the authors also noted the following. 'Parental grief following stillbirth might not be legitimised by health professionals, family and society (disenfranchised grief).' This alarming finding applied to 31 per cent of affected parents, who felt that their loss had been ignored, avoided or minimized. One woman said:

> I went to my GP after I came out of hospital; I was in bits, I was like an automaton. My GP said, 'Look, you and your husband are young, fit and healthy, you just need to get pregnant again and put all this behind you.' I was gobsmacked; she (the GP) just looked at me, gave me one of those smiles and said '... don't worry, you'll soon feel much better'. I just got up and went home, feeling much worse.

Another woman described her experience in hospital after a stillbirth:

> After I had a stillbirth nobody came to ask how I was doing ... doctors and midwives came and went ... they didn't say much ... they did the physical things ... they didn't ask me how I was ... my boyfriend was in tears ... no one spoke to him ... I understand they were very busy and short staffed, but I went home feeling that they didn't care ...

While we hope that these examples do not reflect how the majority of health professionals deal with such tragic situations, they are accounts of women who are reporting events that have occurred in very recent times.

What, then, of the psychological consequences seen by the authors in their collective experience of interviewing, and caring for, hundreds of women and their partners? As noted above, typical accounts provided weeks, months or even many years after the loss describe a very wide range of emotional and other consequences. Rarely does one see individuals who describe a set of symptoms that can be neatly placed into a diagnostic category (for example, major depressive disorder or post-traumatic stress disorder [PTSD]). Having said that, major depression and PTSD are often features of the person's presentation, although these features, almost universally, accompany a wide range of other psychological symptoms, behaviours and wider social effects.

In summary, while research evidence can tell us much about the range of symptoms and the common diagnostic groups that are encountered, there is no such thing as a 'typical case'. Individuals react to this tragedy in their own unique way. In turn, it is our experience that the emotions that follow stillbirth and baby loss often defy description. However, research evidence does assist in obtaining a broad understanding of the consequences and help guide approaches to providing support and coping strategies.

# 2

# Normal and abnormal grief

Overall, when one encounters affected parents, one is touched by the overarching feeling of grief that persists long after the time when a 'normal' bereavement reaction might be expected to fade away. Most of us can remember 'normal grief reactions' when we have been initially shocked and devastated by the loss of a parent, grandparent or best friend. We may be particularly affected by the loss, particularly if it was sudden. In such 'normal' reactions we might also have great difficulty accepting the loss and spend some time experiencing a range of emotions. Nevertheless, for most of us, this reaction is limited in time and very gradually, the intensity of the reaction diminishes. Those of us with religious beliefs might be greatly comforted by the religious rituals that follow death – for example, the funeral mass, the Shiva (in Jewish culture) or, in more secular cultures, the wake or celebration of life. However, the grief that one sees in those affected by stillbirth and perinatal death is, in general, different both in its quantity and quality.

We need to emphasize that, for most parents, even the most intense grief tends to diminish over weeks, or a few months. At the same time, it is true that 'one never forgets'. Even with parents who have eventually coped well and, to some extent, come to terms with the loss, memories will often be triggered many years later, particularly around key times such as anniversary dates, Christmas, Mothers' Day, Fathers' Day and so on. It is not unusual for these parents to also have thoughts 'out of the blue'. For those parents, they need to remember that these memories are a normal and important part of life.

## Prolonged grief

Weeks, months and often years after the event, some parents may continue to experience grief that relentlessly overwhelms each day. In such cases, the loss may not be accepted. In addition,

6

there may be an effect on the ability to relate to others in a normal way, or even to trust family members or friends. Anger, anxiety, emotional numbness and a loss of enjoyment of life are often common features of prolonged grief. These feelings sometimes intensify to the extent that ordinary life grinds to a halt. Although those affected might be able to go back to work or family duties, they might describe themselves as living in their own world and simply 'going through the motions'. Little solace may be provided by the presence of religious rituals, and sometimes there is despair of such a level that they fail to eat properly or care for themselves in the usual way.

One definition of the prolonged grief reaction has been set out in what the *Diagnostic and Statistical Manual of Mental Disorders (DSM-5)* (American Psychiatric Association, 2013), refers to as a persistent complex bereavement-related disorder. The criteria for this outlines that it should follow the death of a close other and that since the death the person should have been experiencing a clinically significant degree of a number of emotions on most days. These emotions can include a persistent yearning for the individual who has been lost, intense sorrow and emotional pain in relation to the death, and a preoccupation with the person who has died and the circumstances surrounding the death.

In addition, the criteria state that the disorder may be diagnosed if the person shows at least six of the following on most days: marked difficulty accepting the death; disbelief or emotional numbness relating to the loss; a difficulty with positively reminiscing about the person who has been lost; bitterness or anger related to the loss; distorted views of oneself in relation to the deceased or the death (for example, self-blaming); an excessive avoidance of anything reminding the person of the loss; a desire to die to be with the person who has been lost; difficulty trusting other people since the death; a feeling of being alone or detached from other people since the death; a feeling that life is meaningless or empty without the one who has died; a belief that the person cannot function without the deceased; confusion about one's role in life or a diminished sense of identity; difficulty with or reluctance to pursue interests or plan for the future (for example, in terms of activities or friends) since the loss; clinically significant distress or an impairment of social, occupational or other important areas of functioning; and the bereavement reaction being out of proportion to or inconsistent with the individual's cultural or religious norms. There are therefore many different combinations of symptoms that may be present, in a sense demonstrating that grief affects people in so many different ways.

Although prolonged grief may respond well to some of the advice provided in this book, or to joining a support organization such as Sands, it is sometimes necessary to seek treatment and care from a health professional. In this case your GP is the obvious first port of call. Part 3 of this book will deal with both self-help and professional approaches.

## PTSD

In addition to feelings of grief, some parents experience many of the signs and symptoms of PTSD. The disorder originates from aspects of the loss that are clearly remembered as being deeply traumatic. Many women recollect the moment when they were told that their baby had died inside them, to which news they reacted with shock, numbness and disbelief. Sometimes, months and years later, they can still see the person breaking that news very clearly, hearing the words in their head and even being able to recall the smells of the room where the news was broken, or the weather outside. Trauma sometimes arises from the experience of sights experienced during labour, delivery and afterwards. Very tragically, for a variety of reasons, the baby's appearance at birth may not be as one might expect, and it is this image that remains in the person's memory. Alternatively, many women and their partners recall the sight of a 'beautiful baby'. However, these memories may also trigger intense distress.

Visual images of these events may occur as 'flashbacks'. Flashbacks can occur at any time, sometimes triggered by seeing a baby in the street, or a television advert for a baby product. Flashbacks are usually very vivid. People sometimes recollect events in 'slow motion' and describe being in a 'blur' and feeling numb. For many, flashbacks often occur as part of a nightmare, waking in a cold sweat, crying and distraught. Even when the memory is of the baby looking, as many have described, as 'beautiful', these images may persist and the sight of the beautiful baby lost may be unbearable.

Flashbacks are often accompanied by more general symptoms, including a depressed mood. The person involved sometimes develops avoidance behaviours that, in some way, remind them of their loss. Other symptoms, such as anger, irritability, mood swings and difficulty getting to sleep, are also very common.

One definition of PTSD is set out in the *Diagnostic and Statistical Manual (DSM-5)* (American Psychiatric Association, 2013). The central requirements for this diagnosis require the affected person to have been exposed to death, threatened death, actual or threatened serious injury, or actual or threatened sexual violence, in one of three ways: by direct exposure, by being a witness to it, or indirectly, by learning that a close relative or close friend has been exposed to trauma. If the event involved actual or threatened death, this must have been violent or accidental. The criteria include events in which professionals or first responders are exposed to diverse events such as collecting body parts or repeated exposure to details of child abuse. However, somewhat controversially, indirect non-professional exposure through electronic media, television, movies or pictures is not included.

The criteria include symptoms occurring in several specific areas, that is, intrusion symptoms in which the traumatic event is persistently re-experienced in one of the following ways: recurrent, involuntary, intrusive memories or traumatic nightmares; disso-ciative reactions (for example, flashbacks); intense or prolonged distress after exposure to reminders of the trauma; or marked physical symptoms, for example palpitations, after exposure to trauma-related stimuli. The criteria also state that there should be evidence that the person is avoiding thoughts or feelings related to the trauma, or external reminders of it (for example, people, places, conversations, activities, objects or situations).

In addition, in this condition people display at least two of the following symptoms affecting thoughts and mood: an inability to recall key features of the traumatic event; persistent (and often distorted) negative beliefs and expectations about oneself or the world (such as 'I am a bad person' or 'The world is utterly dangerous'); a persistent distorted blaming of oneself or others for causing the traumatic event or its consequences; persistent negative emotions about the trauma (for example, fear, horror, anger, guilt and shame); markedly diminished interest in significant activities; a feeling of alienation, for example feeling detached or estranged from others; and a persistent inability to feel positive emotions. The condition may also include irritable or aggressive behavior, self-destructive or reckless behaviour, a heightened awareness of one's environment and being on the look-out for danger, exaggerated physical responses (such as. being very 'jumpy'), and problems with concentration or sleeping. All of the above should have been present for longer than a month and should have caused distress or functional, for example social or occupational, impairment.

Sometimes PTSD occurs immediately, and sometimes it appears many months after the traumatic event.

## PTSD may simply get better without any intervention

It is important to emphasize that countless research studies have shown that even severe PTSD may simply fade away, with flash-backs decreasing in frequency and intensity. Indeed, it is probably important in the first few weeks for professionals not to attempt direct interventions. There is plenty of research showing that interventions that are provided too early on may actually make matters worse. In the early days after loss, emotional support and a very gradual return to 'normal' life and activities are perhaps the most important variables in the beginning of a process aimed at coping and the restoration of 'normal' life.

If you are one of those individuals for whom the PTSD persists, you should try to follow the advice set out later on, in Part 3. If this has little or no effect, it you might require treatment from a professional. Once again, if this is the case, you should discuss this with your GP.

## 'Partial PTSD'

Some women, and sometimes their partners, experience a number of the symptoms described earlier but do not, strictly speaking, meet the full criteria set out above. Nevertheless, in such cases there will be benefit from reading the advice set out in Part 3.

# 3

# Adjustment disorders – panic attacks and persistent memories

For some parents who are suffering very significant levels of distress, their symptoms may not meet the criteria for PTSD or a persistent complex bereavement-related disorder. Instead the symptoms may involve a wide range of great emotional disturbance, including symptoms of anxiety, depression, worry, tension and anger. These may occur in various combinations at different times. These parents are not necessarily suffering less than those who may receive a diagnosis of PTSD; indeed, some parents with the emotional disturbance described above will have some of the symptoms of PTSD – for example, visual flashbacks to the original traumatic events.

The diagnosis applied to parents with a disturbance of emotion described above may be deemed to satisfy the criteria for an 'adjustment disorder'. This is defined in the *International Statistical Classification of Diseases and Related Health Problems*, Version 11 (World Health Organization, 2019). In this classification, an adjustment disorder is defined as a 'maladaptive reaction to an identifiable psychosocial stressor or multiple stressors'. In Part 3 of this book, we will describe in more detail self-help and treatment approaches for the symptoms that form this disorder. However, it is also important to note that adjustment disorders, as with other psychiatric conditions, may gradually improve over time without any professional treatment.

## Avoidance behaviours

Avoidance behaviours are a natural and common phenomenon following stillbirth or perinatal death. If one has been through such a very traumatic episode, one will, quite naturally, be fearful of anything that produces a reminder of that episode. Therefore, in the early days at least, it is common to try to do anything that will avoid reminders of the birth experience, such as the hospital where the event took place, the midwife who comes to visit to support, or those adverts on the television showing happy, bouncing babies. For some, this avoidance can persist and extend to going out on the street, where they might see parents with babies in pushchairs. The sight of healthy babies evokes not only considerable distress, but often intense feelings of anger accompanying the thought, 'Why does that person have a healthy baby and I don't?' Avoidance behaviours may spread to the extent that one's life function becomes impaired and returning to a normal pattern of social activities becomes virtually impossible. Sometimes, even family members and best friends are avoided.

In Part 3 of this book, we will describe a case history (Emma's story) that will highlight the extent of avoidance behaviours that Emma showed and, at the same time, provide some advice about how avoidance behaviours may be combated.

## Hypervigilance and perception of risk

The experience of loss often leads to parents becoming overly aware of potential risks in their environment, and, in one sense, their personality may change from one of being able to put the risks that daily surround us into perspective, to a preoccupation with risk that dominates their life, so that the most remote risk dominates their thinking. Thus, parents often become hypervigilant, that is, they look out everywhere for signs of danger. They may become very anxious about their partner travelling to work; may go into a state of panic when their child develops a minor, common illness; or may imagine all kinds of improbable disasters. Sometimes, in the extreme, this 'risk averseness' leads to not allowing their children to have a babysitter, play with friends or – in some cases we have seen – go to school with other children, so they are then home-schooled.

Hypervigilance is often linked to a lack of trust in others. This is more common in cases where the stillbirth or perinatal death has been attributed to poor standards of care. Therefore, in such cases, there will a loss of trust in all doctors and other health professionals.

## Panic attacks

Panic attacks are very common. Research studies have shown that up to 1 in 3 people have experienced panic during their lifetime. Indeed, in any one year, millions of people in the UK have panic attacks.

The *Diagnostic and Statistical Manual (DSM-5)* (American Psychiatric Association, 2013) sets out the following list of panic symptoms, and states that one needs to experience four or more of them to qualify for the diagnosis of a panic attack. The symptoms usually include many of the following:

- Palpitations
- Sweating
- Trembling or shaking
- Feelings of shortness of breath or smothering
- Feelings of choking
- Chest pain or discomfort
- Feeling sick or having other digestive symptoms
- Feeling dizzy, unsteady, light-headed or faint
- Derealization (feelings of unreality) and depersonalization (feelings of being detached from oneself)
- Fear of losing control
- Fear of dying
- Numbing or tingling sensations
- Chills or hot flushes.

People who have panic attacks have a combination of these symptoms, in various permutations. Many have not just four, but five, six, seven or even all 13 symptoms! Parents who have suffered the loss of a child are very prone to panic attacks, these attacks being triggered by memories of the traumatic event. However, they often come out of the blue. Although people may feel an overwhelming sense of dread when in panic, they are often reassured when told that these symptoms are harmless and caused by the body experiencing a huge surge of arousal in response to stress. In many cases, however, panic attacks develop into a pattern that causes significant distress, with a resultant reduction in quality of life.

Panic attacks are often linked to particular thoughts and triggers. In a sense, panic attacks may be viewed as an amplification of what, for all human beings, is the anxiety that we may suffer from time to time. The anxiety in parents who have suffered loss stems from the individual being in a high state of alert, this high state of alert being maintained by the body's arousal system and the output of the hormone of 'fight or flight,' adrenaline.

We will now set out Ruth's story, describing her first panic attack. In Part 3 of this book (Chapter 13) we will provide an account of Ruth's treatment.

### Case study – Ruth's story, part 1

Ruth gave birth to a baby who had been diagnosed with a problem in the latter part of the pregnancy; this was only discovered, through no one's fault, just weeks before the due date of delivery. Ruth's baby, Jonathan, was born alive but was clearly very unwell and, despite seven days in the paediatric intensive care unit, died in Ruth's arms. Ruth and her partner returned home to their other two children and, in Ruth's words, 'As the grief passed, life went on and we received support from our own parents, brothers and sisters, friends and employers.' After four months, Ruth decided that she should return to full-time work, her employers having given her the option early on of working very restricted hours, which Ruth gratefully accepted. Her boss told her, 'Just see how it goes. Come back full time when you are able.'

On her first day back at work, Ruth decided to go to the local supermarket to buy a sandwich to eat at her desk, as she was quite busy and could not (as was her normal practice) join her friends in the staff canteen. Shortly after Ruth entered the supermarket, she said that she 'didn't feel quite right'. She felt everything was too bright: 'it was all unreal'. She began to feel increasingly unwell and had difficulties breathing. She became very frightened when she felt 'my heart beating out of my chest'. At this point, Ruth dropped her shopping basket and ran out of the supermarket to her office building, just a couple of hundred metres away.

Ruth said that she thought that she was having a heart attack and that she might die, so she ran to her office's reception desk and asked the woman on duty to dial 999. At this point a number of work colleagues came to her assistance and advised that she lie down on the settee in the reception area until the emergency services arrived. By this time Ruth was convinced that she was about to die. Fortunately, a paramedic arrived within a few minutes. At this point Ruth said that she was comforted by this, and later on remarked, 'I knew paramedics can do CPR so, if my heart stopped, he would be able to help.'

After an examination and recording of Ruth's vital signs, the paramedic told her, 'I think you've just had a bad panic attack. However, if you want me to arrange for you to go to hospital, I'll do that.' Ruth accepted this offer and was conveyed to hospital by ambulance. Soon after she arrived in the emergency department, she was feeling physically much better. By this time, Ruth recalls, 'feeling stupid'. After a couple of hours in the emergency department and having been reassured by the ECG results, which showed that her heart was in normal working order, she went home.

Ruth went to see her GP the next day. The GP gave her the last appointment of the day and spent nearly an hour with her. Over the course of the discussion it became clear that Ruth had worried whether her return to work was too soon. She also disclosed to the GP that she had found out on the morning of her return to full-time work that she was going to a meeting at another company; she knew that another woman attending the meeting had just returned to work following the birth of a healthy baby, born around the same time as Jonathan. It thus became clear that the panic attack that Ruth had suffered had been triggered by the apprehension of the day and made worse because its physical symptoms were so frightening. On the GP's advice, Ruth returned to work quite quickly but also attended, following a referral by the GP, a short course of therapy.

## Preoccupation long after the event

Sometimes the preoccupation with loss continues for months, or even years, after the loss. Although, to some extent, much of the grief may diminish, a preoccupation with the loss may involve not only the circumstances of the loss, but also trying to find out why the loss occurred (sometimes an impossible quest). There is often a preoccupation with preventing such a situation happening again, and sometimes the preoccupation becomes so extensive that it blocks out normal family life. The case study that follows will demonstrate another form of preoccupation, albeit in a severe form. In this case the account focuses on an understandable need – to keep the memory of the lost child alive.

### Case study – Roger and Jill's story: a shrine to the lost baby

Roger and Jill began professional treatment three years after the loss of their son, Ryan, who had died minutes after birth. At that time, Roger and Jill had a daughter, Emily (then aged two) and, two years after the loss of Ryan, they had another daughter, Jemma. Roger and Jill were referred because they both had depression that had not really responded to antidepressant medication. The GP noted in her letter of referral that Emily (then aged five years) had demonstrated signs of emotional distress, not wanting to go to school and, despite being, in developmental terms, advanced for her age, bed-wetting every night. Roger and Jill described the feelings of devastation that they had experienced in the aftermath of Ryan's death and how they promised each other that they would never forget him.

Roger and Jill had had one of the bedrooms in their house prepared as a nursery for Ryan. The room had been decorated in colours appropriate for a baby, and the couple had spent a considerable amount of money on furniture, a baby alarm and other items. Ryan was cremated and the couple brought his ashes home in a specially made container, which they put in his cot. They also placed a number of framed pictures of Ryan being cuddled, after his death, by his mother and father around the bedroom. Jill cleaned the room every day, but left everything that had been prepared for his arrival in its place. She and Roger often spent time there, having a cup of tea and talking about how Ryan might have been developing had he lived. Roger decided some months after Ryan's death that he would start running again. He promised that he would devote this activity to raising money in Ryan's name to be given to charities associated with children's deaths. Thereafter, Roger was always in training for a 10k run, a half-marathon or a marathon and had raised literally thousands of pounds in his son's memory to be given to a number of worthy causes.

The couple, being Catholics, frequently attended mass and also, as is the custom in the Catholic religion, had masses said in Ryan's name. However, rather than the custom of most people who might have a mass said once a year, masses were said at different times during the year to coincide with Ryan's birthday, Mothers' Day, Fathers' Day, Easter, Christmas and other occasions.

It became clear at the time of assessment that the lives of Roger and Jill, and their daughters, were dominated by Ryan's memory. When it was put to them that all of these activities might serve to distract from normal family life, they both accepted – at a rational level – that this was so. However, when it was suggested that they might reduce the attention they were giving to Ryan's memory and perhaps begin to think of clearing his nursery, the couple said that they were unable to do this because of feelings of guilt. Indeed, some time before we met, they had decided to reduce the number of masses said in Ryan's name. However, even this small step caused the couple anguish; they felt that they were being disloyal to Ryan. Jill went on to say that she realized that her other two children were, to some extent, not receiving enough attention. She realized that she compensated for this by buying Emily expensive toys and clothes and making a fuss of her. In addition, in keeping with other mothers who have lost children, she described being overprotective to Emily and her younger sister, Jemma.

Eventually, with a small amount of therapy and support from family, friends and their parish priest, the couple were able to regain a balance in their lives. They gradually began to deal with the guilt that they experienced for, in their words, 'not paying Ryan's memory enough attention'. However, they gradually began to see that not engaging in excessive behaviours did not mean that they were being disloyal in any way, and Ryan would always have a special place in their hearts. As time went on, the couple reported that Emily's emotional distress had resolved and the depressions suffered by Roger and Jill had both receded.

We hope that these case studies, and those that follow in this book, will serve to describe the consequences of loss in a way that does more justice than the somewhat 'cold' descriptions found in the classification systems. Perhaps some comfort may also be derived from identifying with the experiences of others.

# 4

# Anger

Feelings of anger are a normal part of bereavement. It is common, in adult life, for people to become angry at the husband or wife who has died, or angry at themselves, because of a feeling that they should have done, or said, something to the deceased. In the case of stillbirth or perinatal death, women often say, 'I'm very angry at myself; I should have done something earlier.' Even when the woman realizes, rationally, that there was nothing that she could have done to alert others, the angry feeling tends to persist. The other parent may also experience angry feelings directed towards themselves and not 'acting sooner' on behalf of the mother.

There is often considerable anger directed towards health professionals for a wide variety of reasons. Sometimes this anger is, to some extent, justified. In many other cases it is not justified. When hospitals conduct investigations they often find that there was nothing that could have been done to prevent the tragedy. For the parents involved, however, anger may grow over a lengthy period because investigations sometimes take many months to complete. In cases where an inquest is held, angry feelings may arise and be maintained by the lengthy delays that are so common within the judicial system. Although, at times, it can be said that anger may be justified, conversely one needs to bear in mind that anger is, primarily, a very destructive emotion. Anger tends to generalize, so that more general irritability occurs and anger may be evoked by relatively trivial events. In Part 3 of this book we will describe strategies that might assist.

### Case study – Joe's story
Joe was born in the Midlands, where he was brought up to enjoy a happy childhood and family life. His one regret while growing up was that he did not have any brothers or sisters. Nevertheless, he had a good group of friends. From an early age Joe wanted to be a police officer and, shortly after leaving school with some 'A' Levels, attended

the police training college. Joe found his life as a police officer very satisfying, and because of his calm and happy demeanour and his skills at interacting with others, his superiors deemed him to be ideal for the role of community policing.

Joe's 'patch' comprised a large housing estate with a great deal of social deprivation. Over the months and then years Joe became a popular figure among the locals. He became involved in the setting up of a number of community activities, including a youth club for boys and girls who would, in the normal course of events, have been left to roam the streets and engage in petty crime. As a police officer, Joe was used to dealing with a very sad part of his job, for example going to houses where someone had died suddenly, or sometimes breaking the bad news of a death. Joe also recalled the way he used to deal with the inevitable insults and taunting that, sadly, have now become part of a police officer's experience. He told me that his colleagues envied him because he was able to defuse many situations by the use of his humour and his calm approach.

Joe met Millie at police training college and the couple became inseparable, eventually marrying at the age of 23. Millie quite quickly became pregnant and gave birth to a healthy boy, whom they called Adam. Millie took long maternity leave and returned to work on a part-time basis, with the assistance of childcare from the couple's respective parents. Millie was also an only child and, like Joe, regretted not having a brother or sister. They therefore looked forward to Millie becoming pregnant again. However, Millie did not fall pregnant quickly and it was only when Adam reached five years of age that Millie was able to break the happy news that she was pregnant again.

Due to Millie being a physically fit young woman, with none of the factors associated with difficulties in pregnancy, she was deemed to be 'low risk'. The pregnancy proceeded well and, at about the due date of delivery, Millie's waters broke. As the intervals between contractions diminished, Joe and Millie went to the maternity unit where she was booked in, leaving Adam behind in the care of his grandparents. Joe, who had been at Adam's birth, was looking forward to the experience of holding his wife's hand during labour and encouraging her with the breathing exercises that she had learned at antenatal classes.

However, late in labour and very suddenly, Millie suffered a massive haemorrhage. This was eventually found to be a condition called a placental abruption, something that could not have been foreseen. Joe was horrified by the sight of Millie haemorrhaging, and even though the doctors and midwives did everything they could, Millie and Joe's baby was born without a pulse. Joe witnessed the frantic efforts at resuscitation and saw the medical team doing everything possible. Sadly, after many minutes, the medical team told Joe that their daughter, who was eventually named Victoria, was dead. By this time, because of the haemorrhage, Millie was unconscious and first needed blood transfusions and then, later on, surgery to stop the bleeding.

Eventually, the couple went home in a state of shock, grateful for the memory box that had been prepared by the midwives. Joe and Millie remained in a state of shock for some time but gradually began to cope with life with the help of a supportive family and the presence of their son, Adam, who had just started school. Millie went back to work fairly quickly and, although very sad and sometimes troubled by 'flashbacks' of the events of that very sad day when Victoria was born, began at last to restart some of the activities she had previously enjoyed outside work.

The story for Joe was very different. Like Millie, Joe was troubled by flashbacks and what could be described as a heart-rending bereavement process. However, while Millie's grief began to ebb away, the emotion that came to dominate Joe's life was that of anger. Joe later said that he could not understand why he was angry or who he was angry at. He acknowledged that the doctors and midwives had done everything they could and had exercised a great deal of skill. After Victoria's death, the midwives and doctors showed very comforting compassion.

Joe found himself becoming angry at all kinds of things: turning on the television and hearing news of the latest terrorist attack caused him to become uncharacteristically extremely angry, and he would find himself kicking doors and furniture. When he went back to work, situations that he had previously managed by his calm demeanour began to irritate him and, rather than speaking quietly to defuse a situation at work, he found himself raising his voice and being very abrupt with members of the general public. Joe realized that his level of anger was interfering with his job, but did not know what to do.

One day, on his way to work, another driver 'cut him up'. Joe reacted with 'road rage,' something that had never happened before, and he drove behind the driver who had caused the incident, flashing his lights, blaring the horn and making obscene signs. When Joe calmed down he realized that his anger was becoming out of control. He decided to visit his GP, who had known him for many years.

Joe's GP recognized that Joe needed some professional help and advised him to take some sick leave. Joe was referred to the counsellor attached to the GP practice; however, there was a long waiting list. Fortunately, the occupational adviser attached to the police service arranged for Joe to obtain an earlier appointment. The therapist that Joe saw took three sessions, each one hour long, to make an assessment of Joe's problems. It became clear that Joe had, to a large extent, 'bottled up' some of the emotions caused by the events surrounding his daughter's birth and death. Although he had shared some of his emotions with Millie and others, he had kept to himself his horrified reaction to the sight of Millie bleeding, and the source of his anger appeared to be caused by his question, 'Why?'

The therapist wisely suggested that Joe kept a diary to monitor his thoughts and feelings. This strategy appeared to put Joe more in control, as he came to realize that certain thoughts triggered angry feelings. The therapist also suggested that Joe learned some methods to deal with anger, notably the use of breathing and meditation techniques. At first Joe was somewhat dismissive of meditation, but after some encouragement from the therapist, he downloaded a meditation app on to his phone and came to realize that using the skills acquired during meditation might assist him to defuse his anger.

Joe was off work for six weeks and, on the advice of his occupational health adviser, began a phased return to work, initially confining himself to working in the police station rather than going out on to the streets. On his return to work Joe found out that his boss, a Superintendent, had also experienced a stillbirth, and he told Joe his own story. This disclosure helped Joe a great deal. Because his superintendent had some understanding of Joe's troubles, he put in place more detail of a phased return to work, including increasing Joe's exposure to the public in small steps.

Joe had six more meetings with his therapist over the following six months. In these meetings the therapist suggested ways of coping with other aspects of Joe's emotional turmoil and, gradually, Joe's anger subsided. A year after the couple's tragedy, Joe said that although he would never return to how he was before, he had regained much of his previous personality and outlook. As for Millie, a year after the loss of Victoria, she said that providing Joe with help and support was something that seemed to benefit her. Once Joe became more open about all of his feelings, Millie said that she and Joe's love for each other had intensified and made their marriage stronger.

## Increased use of alcohol and the use of other drugs

Some parents deal with their loss by self-medication, often using drugs such as cannabis to alleviate their anxiety and increase their feelings of well-being. Alcohol use may increase. However, both substance use and alcohol inevitably worsen the problems because of the negative consequences associated with problem drinking or intoxication with illicit substances.

In general, traumatic events are associated with a consequent increase in the use of alcohol. Many parents say that their alcohol use increased for a period after their loss. However, many recognize that this increase in alcohol is not helpful and that the short-term relief that obtained after a few drinks is then replaced by a depressive mood.

One very helpful and simple way of determining if you have a problem with alcohol is to use the Michigan Alcohol Screening Test. This is available on the internet at no charge – see <www.counsellingresource.com/lib/quizzes/drug-testing/alcohol-mast/>. An alternative, universally used self-administered test is FAST, which detects whether drinking is hazardous. This is a four-item questionnaire that asks:

1  How often you have had eight or more drinks?
2  How often in the past year have you been unable to remember?
3  How often during the past year have you failed to do what is normally expected of you because of your drinking?
4  Has a friend or relative, a doctor or other health worker been concerned about your drinking or suggested that you cut it down?

Details of the FAST questionnaire may be found at: https://assets. publishingservice.giv.uk/6357a7ebe90e0777aa2cfe96.

Individuals with PTSD are very susceptible to the use of alcohol and drugs. Sadly, illicit drugs are widely available and are to some extent, as in the case of cannabis, gaining increasing public approval; in some parts of the world the laws concerning drug use are becoming more relaxed.

Professionals face the difficulty of making a correct assessment of the extent of alcohol or substance use in those who come to us for help. We are therefore in their hands and need to depend on their honesty in telling us what substances they use, how much they use and what effects these have. Sometimes the matter of honesty is not entirely straightforward because people – particularly those who are developing alcohol dependency problems – have ways of denying the extent of the problem to themselves.

Sadly, traumatic events often result in destructive emotions and behaviours. In the great majority of people we have encountered who have experienced such loss, anger, either directed at others or more internalized, is an emotion of significant proportions. As the later sections of this book will demonstrate, there are various helpful strategies that may be employed. In turn, the harmful use of drugs and alcohol will often diminish once these negative emotions are subjected to coping strategies.

# 5

# Effects on relationships

There may be substantial effects on the parents' relationship. Sometimes loss brings parents together and past difficulties in their relationships are put to one side. Conversely, it is quite common for such a loss to cause a breakdown in what may have been a previously good relationship – this breakdown, sadly, sometimes becoming permanent. We will, in Part 3 of this book, provide some advice on dealing with the problems in relationships that might arise.

*Case study – Linda and Roy's story*
Linda and Roy met when they were both 22 years of age and lived together for three years before they married at the age of 26. When they married they took a conscious decision to delay having children until they were 30 years old, so they could save for a new house and progress their careers in the meantime. This, they decided, was so that when a baby came along, Linda could have a possibility of going back to work part time.

Linda described their lives up to the tragic event as 'charmed'. Both had loving families and good social networks. They were a hard-working couple, who also enjoyed active participation in sports (Linda was a runner and Roy played football). They both enjoyed a drink with their friends at weekends, although they did not drink alcohol during the week. Neither Linda nor Roy smoked, and both were in excellent physical health. By the time that Linda became pregnant with Melanie-Anne – a name derived from much-loved aunts in Linda's and Roy's families – they described themselves as 'much in love'. Of particular relevance, they had always enjoyed the physical intimacy of their marriage.

Apart from some early morning sickness, Linda's pregnancy was ideal. She did not put on too much weight, and she worked until she was 36 weeks' pregnant (by this time feeling a little tired). Both her obstetrician and her midwife reassured Linda that she was in 'great shape', and the various prenatal examinations and scans showed a normal pregnancy with Melanie-Anne developing without any problems.

Linda went into labour and all seemed to be going well. She eventually presented to the local hospital, where she was booked in and labour appeared to proceed smoothly. However, for reasons that are still unknown, Melanie-Anne's heartbeat decreased and a decision was made to perform an emergency caesarean section under general anaesthetic; the general anaesthetic was required because the doctors and midwives formed the view that the baby needed to be delivered as soon as possible.

Linda described how the few minutes between Melanie-Anne's condition deteriorating and the anaesthetic being delivered were 'a complete blur'. Linda says that she remembers coming around from the anaesthetic and asking where Melanie-Anne was. At this point she said that she saw Roy's face and the face of one of the midwives and immediately knew that Melanie-Anne had died. Linda then said, 'I knew she was dead, but I didn't believe it. I was in a state of shock and numbness … '.

Linda then said that she remembers screaming, and again everything became somewhat of a blur. Linda recollected that in the days before she was discharged, all she could remember was the sound of babies crying in other parts of the ward – she was in one of the side rooms. Linda did not want to see any visitors and wanted to just hang on to Roy. She remembers that he, too, was distraught, and they barely said a word to each other.

Eventually, when it came to Linda's discharge from hospital, Linda and Roy returned to Linda's parents' home as neither of them could contemplate facing their own home again with a newly decorated nursery full of the sort of contents that would remind them of Melanie-Anne. Linda said that it was at this point that she clearly recollects 'a wall building' between herself and Roy; they were barely able to say more than a few words to each other and, for reasons that neither could explain, became argumentative, usually over very trivial matters. Eventually, following Melanie-Anne's funeral, they returned to their own house, but the wall between them seemed, in Linda's own words, to grow and solidify.

Although they both returned to work, they avoided virtually all interactions outside the immediate family. Linda was able to speak to her mother, father and brother, but avoided seeing her sister, who had two young children, one of whom was a nine-month-old baby. Linda said that any contact with her sister made her angry, as did the sight of women in the street wheeling their babies along in prams and buggies. In addition to her job, Linda threw herself into domestic activity and, instead of spending a reasonable period of time on household chores, began to clean obsessively and found herself shopping, buying things that she had no use for.

All Roy's energy went into his work and he became more and more distant. Before Melanie-Anne's birth, Roy had enjoyed cooking and had done his fair share of cleaning and gardening. The couple's 'weekly shop' was a very pleasant event where they engaged in light-hearted banter and usually concluded with a pub lunch, or a trip to the cinema or a sporting event. All this stopped; if Roy was not at work, he brought work home with him and was focused on his job seven days a week, with no time for anything else. Although there was no physical reason to explain this, Linda and Roy did not resume any physical intimacy apart from one, isolated episode six months after Melanie-Anne's death.

Both Linda and Roy went to their GP. Roy was prescribed some sleeping tablets and offered counselling, which he refused. Linda similarly refused counselling, but accepted an antidepressant medication, which she began but stopped after two weeks because she said she could not tolerate the side effects. Linda described their marriage at this point as follows.

> We were like two strangers, living in the same house. We were civil to each other, but not able to tolerate more than a few minutes of each other's presence. Other people tried to get us to talk. With the benefit of hindsight, we were both preoccupied about the loss of Melanie-Anne, but could not communicate this to each other, or indeed to anyone else ... Roy avoided thinking or talking about Melanie-Anne ... I did the same by a number of useless activities.

Linda and Roy separated after 18 months and divorced three years after Melanie-Anne's death. Linda sought psychiatric treatment for her depression. It was only then that she began to talk openly about her loss. By then she had only minimal contact with Roy, who had moved to another part of the country and had, according to Linda, 'thrown himself into work and was a completely different man from the one I married'.

This story illustrates the sometimes devastating consequences for a marriage following the loss of a child. Such apparently extreme reactions to the loss of a child often defies explanation. In the case of Linda and Roy, there was absolutely no history of any mental health problems and, objectively, they had, prior to Melanie-Anne's death, what many would describe as an ideal marriage.

## Effects on sexual relationships

The loss of a baby often causes a breakdown in a sexual relationship between the parents. However, there are many other causes of sexual difficulties for parents: low mood and depression very often lead to a great reduction in sexual interest and, quite simply, a preoccupation with depressing thoughts leaves little else to think about. At this point we must mention that there may be physical reasons for problems with sexual activity. Sometimes the woman has suffered an injury during childbirth that may be the cause. Very sadly, some women are too embarrassed to seek medical help, and the problems persist. We strongly advise that, if this is the case, it is very important that you consult your GP. Such problems will be very familiar to them, and most problems like this will respond to treatment.

Sometimes attempts at sexual activity trigger thoughts of the whole process of conception, pregnancy and birth, so sexual intimacy is avoided. Another common problem that arises is that of anxiety affecting normal sexual physiology. For the man this may lead to difficulties with erection or premature ejaculation; the woman may suffer an involuntary spasm of the vaginal muscles that makes intercourse painful or impossible. Sexual difficulties in men and woman often lead to a pattern of avoiding sexual activity because of a fear of failure. In Part 3 of this book we will describe simple methods that may help parents overcome some of these problems.

# 6

## Other effects

### Effects on future pregnancies

Parents often go on to have more children. However, although becoming pregnant is usually a happy experience, the new pregnancy may be a 'bittersweet experience' for those who have suffered loss. Many women describe never being reassured by normal scans, or by the reassurance provided by health professionals. They may engage in excessive checking for signs of miscarriage or, later on, of abnormal fetal movement.

When another child is born, this too can also become a 'bittersweet experience' because a healthy, smiling baby triggers reminders. In such situations, parents often say 'I wonder what (the lost child) would make of his/her brother/sister?' In turn, the sight of other children, born at the same time as the occurrence of the stillbirth or perinatal death, will trigger thoughts of how that child might have been now. One woman said, 'I try to work out how she would have turned out. I even rehearse in my mind how I might deal with teenage rebellion ... '.

### Effect on employment

Employment may suffer as a consequence of stillbirth or perinatal death. This may be because of a disinclination to go back to work; this disinclination being triggered by the thought that one would need to mix with parents and pregnant women, and this in turn, might trigger more distress. Conversely, it is common to see women and their partners 'throw themselves into work' as an attempt to cope with loss. Such behaviours (described above in the case of Linda and Roy) often serve to further damage relationships that may have been affected by avoidance.

We all need to balance our lives. Although there is a need to work, whether that be at home or going to an outside job, we also need to enjoy time with the family and take part in enjoyable activities, ranging from dinner out or a trip the cinema to attending a sporting event and so on. In Part 3 of this book we will say more about employment and provide some advice about a topic that causes many substantial difficulties.

## The effect of stillbirth and perinatal death on health professionals

This topic is not given much space in the substantial number of publications available on stillbirth and perinatal death. Nevertheless, we can speak from our own experience by saying that witnessing stillbirth or listening to accounts of stillbirth may be deeply distressing for the professionals involved. As a professional, one is meant to recognize the distress in others but, all too often, one is also told, 'This is part of the job ... you just have to learn to get used to it.' Such advice does not take account of the simple fact that all professionals are also human and react to the suffering of others in differing ways.

The authors of this book have had the experience of witnessing death and dying in their many forms. We both agree that the effect of witnessing the suffering of others may be cumulative. Both of us will also tell you that events of 30 years or more ago remain clearly in our minds and sometimes, without warning, we will recall these events – sometimes with vivid visual imagery. With regard to stillbirth, *The Lancet* review (see Chapter 1), described the psychological effect of stillbirth on professionals, citing research that 95 per cent of professionals say it has a powerful psychological effect and may result in emotional response or distancing, trauma and guilt. Sometimes these feelings of guilt are irrational – driven by the thoughts 'Could I have done something different? Did I miss something?' These thoughts often persist even when there is no rational basis for them. In our experience, anger is another emotion that arises not because anyone has done anything wrong, but from the question, 'Why has this happened to such a lovely person?'

Different professionals experience emotions in different ways, depending on their particular role. Midwives may be affected by many things – the sight of a stillborn child, dealing with a woman who is inconsolable, or being so busy that their own distress is never expressed because there is so much to do. One very experienced midwife described how she was 'ashamed' at being so upset and could only retreat to the lavatory so that she could shed her tears. Psychologists may be affected because they listen to very many graphic descriptions, often for lengthy periods of time. In the course of therapy, they will hear these descriptions many times over.

There is now increasing recognition that health professionals and, indeed, other people involved in helping roles, such as police officers, paramedics and firefighters, need emotional support and, sometimes, professional treatment. One of the most common methods of ensuring that health professionals and others do not suffer adverse psychological consequences is the 'group debrief'. This involves professionals and their peers discussing the traumatic event and, through a process of sharing and support from colleagues, defusing some of the toxic emotional reactions. Sadly, although many services use this approach extensively, there are still parts of the health service where its use is somewhat restricted.

## When things could have been done better

Sadly, a small proportion of stillbirths and perinatal deaths should not have happened. Had a reasonable level of care been provided, a healthy baby would have been born and survived. There are many causes of such events. Sometimes the warning signs that indicate a substantial problem have been missed; sometimes there is a problem with the way in which labour and delivery are managed. In some instances there may not be sufficient numbers of adequately trained health professionals available to deal with a problem when it arises. In such cases the hospital is under an obligation to conduct an investigation to establish the facts.

Sadly, the investigation process may take weeks or even months to complete. Investigations may involve considering the results of a post mortem, conducting interviews with all those involved and seeking the services of an independent professional. This individual can look at the circumstances without any bias – because they are not employed by the hospital. Thus, the investigation itself may add yet another very stressful factor on top of what is obviously a grave loss to the parents.

It must be said that, sometimes, when it appears at first sight that things have gone wrong that should not have gone wrong, the investigation shows that the stillbirth or death could not have been prevented. It may also be shown that the professionals involved did all that they could in those particular circumstances. As we have described at the beginning of this book, there are so many reasons why stillbirth and perinatal death occur and, sometimes, due to the complexity, it is very difficult to see what exactly went wrong.

There are now a significant number of cases where the parents have sued (or are in the process of suing) the NHS. Although we would not wish in any way to provide advice about whether to take this step, all we can say is that, from our experience, legal claims themselves can be very stressful and take months or years to complete. Both authors have experience of such cases and we know that, to their credit, the solicitors involved will make very clear that taking a claim forward is a serious matter that requires a great deal of thought and discussion.

Unfortunately, in cases where things have gone wrong, anger is the prevailing emotion if parents come to believe that their loss could have been prevented by a reasonable standard of care. In addition, failures by health professionals may lead to the parents developing a more general distrust of health professionals, and future pregnancies will be much feared. If and when a woman becomes pregnant again, she sometimes feels that she cannot return to the same hospital or service in which the loss occurred, even if this is local and convenient for her. In such cases, women are generally treated with a great deal of care and consideration, and there should be no problems associated with transferring their care, if that is what is thought best, to another hospital or service.

The doctors and midwives involved in future pregnancies should be very mindful of the natural fear and apprehension involved on the part of the parents. It has been our experience that, in such cases, it is helpful to arrange for additional antenatal scans and more regular appointments with the doctors and midwives.

# Part 2
# A MIDWIFERY PERSPECTIVE AND SOME FACTS

# 7

# The role of midwives

Midwifery is one of the very oldest professions, being first referred to in the Bible (Exodus 1:15–21), when the King of Egypt told the Hebrew midwives to kill all the babies at birth if they were male. Happily, the midwives did not follow the orders and as a result the Bible tells us, 'God dealt well with the midwives.' However, centuries were to pass before midwifery became the accepted profession it is today.

It first received legal recognition in 1902, when the English Midwives Act was passed and the Central Midwives Board set up to regulate the training and practice of midwives. In 1936 another Midwives Act was passed that made it compulsory for every local authority to employ sufficient midwives to care for all the child-bearing women in their area. However, it was not until the NHS came into effect in 1948 that midwives were provided free of charge to all women.

Since the broadcast of television programmes such as *Call the Midwife* and *One Born Every Minute*, the general public are probably more aware today of the midwife's role than they previously have been. However, they may not fully realize the extent of the role and how the NHS relies on them for providing the majority of care to women during pregnancy, birth and the postnatal period, and also for the care of newborn babies. Registered midwives are the accepted experts in normal child-birth and they can, when there are no complications, undertake the total care of pregnant women, deliver their babies and provide care for the mother and her baby in the postnatal period. All this can be done without referral to a doctor. Therefore, in the UK it is accepted that midwives are the main caregivers of women during childbirth. Although the rate of caesarean sections has risen steeply in recent times, and as a result many obstetricians now deliver babies, over half of all the babies born in the UK are still delivered by midwives.

For many years, midwives have been responsible for undertaking additional work that was not traditionally considered part of their role. This includes a type of surgery (called an episiotomy) when required, which makes a small cut at the entrance to the vagina to make more room for the baby to be born, and undertaking suturing to repair any cuts or tears. Midwives have also been trained to resuscitate newborn babies to a standard on a par with paediatricians of house officer status. When complications arise, midwives can make direct referrals to obstetricians and other professionals, and summon paediatricians to babies. They can also work alongside anaesthetists, topping up epidurals in labour. When complications arise the midwives are also responsible for monitoring the condition of mothers and their unborn babies, and they are the workforce undertaking the treatment planned by obstetricians, paediatricians and anaesthetists. Midwives can also work in theatre, passing instruments to the obstetricians during caesarean sections and, when required, assist paediatricians when babies require advanced means of resuscitation. After qualification, some midwives choose to work in neonatal units which involves specializing in providing care for sick and pre-term babies.

In recent times the midwife's role has extended further than this and it now encompasses the ability to prescribe some medicines and undertake ultrasound scanning during pregnancy. Midwives can now also undertake a full examination of the baby before he or she goes home, which is a role that was previously undertaken by a paediatrician. Therefore, every woman in the UK who becomes pregnant will receive all or part of her care from a midwife, and for this reason midwives are the professionals who are fundamentally involved with parents when the loss of a baby occurs.

Midwives' training is full time and can take three years. Training consists of integrated theory and clinical practice. Theory is provided in universities, and the clinical experience takes place in different settings, such as the community, maternity units in hospitals and birth centres. During their training, student midwives, like their European counterparts, are required to provide antenatal care for at least 100 pregnant women. They are also required to take part in parent education, informing women of the choices they can make regarding the place of birth, prepare women for labour and provide information on the types of pain relief that are available in the different settings. They also give women information on breast-feeding and the care of the baby after delivery.

Student midwives must observe at least ten normal deliveries and provide care for at least 40 labouring women, including personally delivering the baby. In addition to this, they care for women having epidural blockades, in which pain-blocking drugs are injected into the space surrounding the spinal cord, but at the same time allow the woman to 'bear down' and experience contractions. In addition, student midwives also assist obstetricians during instrumental deliveries and caesarean sections. They also are required to provide care for at least 100 women and their babies after the birth. During their training they spend a short time working in a neonatal unit, caring for sick and pre-term babies.

Midwifery training focuses on three main areas – pregnancy, labour/delivery and the postnatal period – which also includes the care of the baby following birth. Students learn first about normal childbirth, and then about various complications that can arise during pregnancy, labour or birth and in the postnatal period. Although students learn the theory of complications that can arise and their management in the university, it is during their clinical placements that they gain first-hand experience of these complications and how to develop a management plan.

Each year of training is carefully assessed, ensuring both theoretical and practical competence. There are also final examinations at the end of training; these include both written and oral assessments. On successful completion of the course the student midwife is registered with the UK Nursing and Midwifery Council (NMC) and is awarded the title of Registered Midwife (RM). The NMC is responsible for regulating all Registered Nurses and Midwives in the UK. At the end of March 2018 there were 690,278 nurses and midwives on the NMC register.

Like any newly qualified individual, midwives are of course relatively inexperienced, and their wisdom and knowledge can only be increased through further experience. Indeed, midwives receive regular training updates to ensure that they maintain sufficient continuing professional development.

It was established many years ago that there is a shortage of midwives. This can obviously put babies lives at risk (Ashcroft et al., 2003). Current publications from the Royal College of Midwives (RCM) report there has been no improvement in numbers, despite early warnings. A report by the RCM in 2017 (RCM, 2107a) calculated that, in England, the NHS had a shortfall equivalent to 3,500 full-time midwives. However, figures show that, conversely, there is a rising trend in the number of births, as in the 12 months leading up to 31 March 2016 there were almost 11,500 more births than in the previous year (RCM, 2017a).

Another report by the RCM (RCM, 2016a) confirmed that, in addition to the rising birth rate, more women were delaying childbearing until they were older. The report confirmed that, since 2001, there had been an increase of more than 12,000 births to women over the age of 40. At the same time, it is known that older women have a higher rate of complications. In addition to this problem, the RCM reported that more than one in five pregnant women in England and Scotland were obese (that is, 21 per cent and 22 per cent, respectively), obesity being known to increase the rate of complications. When women have complications, more demands are placed on maternity services, in turn producing a corresponding need for more midwives.

In December 2017, the RCM published a news statement reporting the findings of a survey involving heads of midwifery services (RCM, 2017c). It was estimated that half of the maternity units had to close their doors to labouring women in the previous year because they were unable to cope with the demand. Forty-nine per cent of the heads of midwifery services surveyed reported that they had to close their doors at least once due to serious concerns over safety. One unit had to close its doors due to understaffing and fears for safety 33 times during 12 months. In total, units closed 209 times, with an average of six closures per unit and six units closed on ten or more occasions.

Increased demands were caused by the number of complex pregnancies/births and low midwifery staffing levels. Over a third of the heads of midwifery services actually reported that they did not have enough midwives to cope with the demands of the service, and that the demands in 2016 were significantly higher than they had been in the previous year. Notwithstanding this, the heads of midwifery reported that their budgets for maternity services had been cut from the previous year, and these cuts had caused some of the services they provided (such as parent classes, breast-feeding support and bereavement support) to be reduced (RCM, 2016b). This example clearly demonstrates how the quality of care can be influenced by the constraints that maternity units face. The general public are often unaware of such problems.

The difficulties units face also have direct consequences for midwives. In 2017 the RCM reported that the shortage of midwives was causing a vicious cycle, with many midwives leaving the profession altogether. Almost half of the RCM members surveyed in March 2016 reported that they felt stressed virtually every day, and the reason they gave was the increased size of their workload (RCM, 2017a). They cited midwifery shortages as a main reason for their stress, as well as the fact that they did not have enough time to spend with women for providing the care they felt they ought to provide. They concluded by stating that the three main reasons for leaving the profession were increased workload or responsibilities, lack of staff and not having enough time to provide care (RCM, 2017a).

However, it seems unlikely that this situation will improve, as another survey published by the RCM in 2017 (RCM, 2017b) reported that midwives involved in teaching also described feeling stressed, due to heavy workloads in the universities, particularly those involving paperwork and administration. This caused them to work a significant number of unpaid extra hours to meet the demands. They also faced additional pressure from universities to publish research and gain extra qualifications. As a result, many reported that they planned to leave within two years. If this occurs it may well result in an insufficient number of lecturers to teach the next generation of midwives.

Since September 2017 the number of applications to train as a midwife has dropped significantly in one leading teaching university. In addition, previous applicants involved a significant number of mature women with life experiences, their own children and the ability to identify with labouring women. Applicants now, however, are mainly 18-year-old college leavers with the ability to obtain student loans.

This has followed the decision to cut the bursary awards given to student midwives during their training. Instead applicants now have to pay the universities £9,000 a year to train as a midwife, in addition to working a 37½ hour week (involving unsociable working hours) during clinical placements. Unless this decision is reversed it is likely to create a future negative impact on the number and experience of midwives working in the NHS. In addition, as one in three midwives currently working in England are now in their fifties or sixties, many of them are set to retire soon (RCM, 2016a). This will lead to a reduction in the number of experienced midwives, in turn likely to affect the standard of care that can be provided.

Conversely, obstetricians are experts in abnormal or complicated childbirth and therefore they are the professionals responsible for women who have existing medical conditions or obstetric problems. In such cases obstetricians plan the care, some of which they also carry out, but some is also undertaken by midwives, who assist at instrumental deliveries and caesarean sections. Even with the best possible care, however, it should be remembered that it is not possible to save all babies. Sadly, it is also true that some babies might have survived if different action had been taken at the time. The hurt produced by such a possibility often results in claims of negligence being made by the families.

Sadly, our legal system is adversarial, which means that bringing a claim for negligence can be very upsetting and traumatic for the parents and their family. However, they may feel vindicated in fighting for their lost child and it might also prevent the loss of other babies.

# 8

# A midwife's perspective

As a midwife, I have cared for many women over the years who have lost a baby, as either a stillbirth, a neonatal death or a sudden infant death. I will never forget any of them, despite the passage of time. I am also aware that the families involved never forget the babies. Although a midwife primarily aims his or her care at the mother, he or she also has to consider other family members when a baby dies, because it affects the whole family, including other children and grandparents. The loss of a baby before, or soon after, birth, leaves a wound that is difficult to heal. Even if the mother becomes pregnant again, the memory of what happened and the fear of reoccurrence will never be far away, for herself or her family. A comparison often occurs between each stage of a new pregnancy or the next baby's early life, and there is fear of recurrence until the same stage has passed.

This was brought home to me one very busy night shift, many years ago, when I was providing care for a labouring woman who had previously had two stillbirths. The woman and her husband were very anxious, as the two previous babies had both died shortly before birth. During the night, it became apparent that the mother required a caesarean section, due to signs of fetal distress. Although there were no immediate concerns for the baby, the mother had a general anaesthetic, which meant that her husband was not allowed in theatre with her. It was a very busy night shift and I tried to reassure both parents. However, as we were going into theatre, I remember the father sitting alone outside. I will never forget the look of terror on his face, or the sheer panic in his voice. Until the baby was born and both his wife and baby were safe, nothing I said could alleviate this.

## Management of loss in the past and today

In the past the care given to parents losing a baby was very different from what it is today. When I qualified as a midwife in 1974 my training did not include how to respond to mothers having a stillbirth or neonatal death. As a result, these tragedies were very often handled quite poorly.

At that time many of the routine antenatal screening tests we now take for granted were unavailable. Therefore babies were sometimes born with unexpected serious abnormalities, causing a shock for both the mother and the midwife. Some of the problems were incompatible with life and the baby was either stillborn or lived for only a very short time. In those early days, stillborn babies or those dying soon after birth were not usually given to their mothers or fathers to hold; instead everything was managed in a clinical way. As a result, parents were deprived of memories of the baby, sometimes not even knowing what the baby looked like, and the baby was often not given a name. Contrary to what was thought best at the time, such practice did not make the loss of the baby any easier for the family to bear.

In the past, I and many other midwives, who did not have bereavement training, could find caring for a mother who had lost a baby very difficult. As a community midwife I recall the apprehension I experienced about meeting a mother in our local town who had lost a baby. This apprehension was caused by feelings of inadequacy and of not knowing what to say or do. However, one experience taught me that it was very important, when seeing mothers and their families, to acknowledge their loss and show my own sadness.

There is one experience that I will never forget. This involved a mother who had lost a baby through sudden infant death syndrome (SIDS) at six weeks of age. When I heard about it I was devastated, as I had got to know the family well during the pregnancy and after the birth. The family even had a picture of me bathing the baby. When the mother became pregnant again she specifically asked for me as her named midwife. I was quite apprehensive about going to see her for the first time. However, she was so pleased to see me that she immediately put me at ease.

I felt very humble to be on the receiving end of her comfort, rather than her being on the receiving end of mine. I realized afterwards that she found seeing me a comfort, not distressing (which I thought would be the case because it would bring back painful memories of her loss). Our meeting brought back some happy memories of the baby she had been able to keep for only a short time, and these moments were very precious to her.

Over the years it has gradually become clear that midwives need to be given some form of training to prepare them for dealing sensitively with parents and families when a baby dies. In 2010 the Royal College of Obstetricians and Gynaecologists (RCOG, 2010b) developed guidelines for healthcare professionals for this purpose, and student midwives are now taught how to deal sensitively with the loss of a baby during their training. However, there is no standardized national training, and any training is usually organized and provided at a local level by a linked university. The need to provide information for bereaved families was also recognized by the RCOG. In July 2012 they issued a booklet for parents who had lost a baby (RCOG, 2012a). Since then the charity Sands has produced its own national guidelines for professionals; this includes recommendations from the National Institute of Health and Clinical Excellence (NICE) and other Royal Colleges and it is now in its fourth edition (Sands, 2016a).

Sands also provides standardized bereavement training for student midwives, qualified midwives, other healthcare professionals and also lay people. Midwives who feel specially drawn to work in the area of bereavement can attend this training and specialize in the role of 'bereavement midwife' for their local NHS Trust, supporting women and their families after loss. However, the availability of bereavement midwives varies between the different NHS Trusts, as larger maternity hospitals may have more than one bereavement midwife (who may not necessarily work full time). However, smaller maternity units may not have any, or may have only one who works part time. Therefore there is considerable variation in the availability of bereavement support provided by hospitals. As we have noted before, many charities provide individual support for bereaved parents and support groups. At the end of the book is a list of the names and addresses of some of these.

I have seen great changes over the years in the manner in which families and their lost babies have been treated. Change began when midwives started to take photographs of the baby for the family and, if possible, a lock of hair. If the parents found it too upsetting to keep these items, they were kept inside the mother's case notes, so that they could be given to the parents later if they changed their mind. Following on from this, handprints and footprints were also taken and given to the parents, or kept in the notes for later.

The charity Sands now provides a memory box for every family losing a baby, whether before birth, during birth or after birth. Examples of a memory box given by Sands include, for example, a memory box tied with ribbon and containing a hand-knitted or crocheted blanket and two teddy bears. One teddy stays with the baby and the other remains in the box for the parents. There is also a small gossamer-type butterfly bag to keep a lock of the baby's hair in. Parents can of course create their own box with their own personal mementos. In addition, Sands provides a handprint and footprint kit, so that parents can take their own baby prints and create their own memories. There is also a card to keep the prints on.

The Sands booklet entitled 'Saying goodbye to your baby' provides information for parents on many issues, including emotional and physical reactions to grief and practical information on such topics as registration, funerals and financial benefits parents may be entitled to. Another booklet, entitled 'Footprints', contains a collection of stories and poems for parents, which shares the experiences and thoughts of other bereaved parents and their families.

Sands also provide parents with a Family Support Pack (Sands, 2016b), which contains booklets giving information about their service. Further booklets in it include one entitled 'Saying goodbye to your baby'. Others contain information mainly for fathers, information and support for grandparents, support for other children, for other family and friends, and on late miscarriage. Sands also provides information for deciding about a post mortem, a funeral, returning to work after the death of a baby, sexual relations after the death of a baby and embarking on another pregnancy. Information for employers is available too.

Other charities also provide some items for the parents, which enables them to keep precious memories. Some may give a SIM card for a mobile phone so the family can take photographs. A Moses basket can sometimes be lent to the family and baby clothes given, even for the smallest of babies. I know of a local group of women who knit the tiniest baby clothes and donate them to the local neonatal unit, where they are used for babies on the unit and also given to families of very small babies who have died.

When a baby has been stillborn or died in hospital, most maternity units have a self-contained quiet family room for bereaved parents, away from the noise of crying babies. The mother and father can remain in this room for the duration of the hospital stay. The room will contain a double bed and drink-making facilities, and food can be obtained from the ward. The baby can stay with them in a 'cold cot', which is kept refrigerated. The length of stay in hospital is at the parents' discretion, but it might also depend on the mother's condition and whether she requires further treatment. Most parents decide to go home from hospital as soon as possible, rather than remaining in a place that holds upsetting memories. However, going home can also involve heartache: the bereavement trainer from Sands has told us how parents report that going home with 'empty arms' can even produce a physical ache.

If parents choose to do so, they can take their baby home with them in a cooled cot, lent to them by the hospital. This helps to keep the baby fresh and allow all members of the family, including grandparents and other extended family members, to spend time with the baby and have photographs taken. I recall one family who took their stillborn baby home for four days prior to the funeral. During this time the baby (who had been given a name before his birth), was photographed and held by all members of the family, including his older brother. This enabled him to be spoken to and talked about by name, and treasured as an individual family member. After the funeral, the memories and the mementos they collected enabled him to be remembered in a similar manner to other family members who had passed away.

Nowadays, society's value for lost babies is apparent by the manner in which we treat them after death and in the funerals, cremations and gardens of remembrance specifically designed for babies. This is a great contrast to the distant past, when parents were not encouraged to speak about, or remember, their lost baby.

They were even encouraged to forget the date of the baby's birth or death, and not memorialize it. As a result, grief was stifled, but, contrary to what was intended, this did not make bearing the loss any easier and the babies were still never forgotten. In the personal experience of one of the authors, even at the end of the mother's life, she never forgot the baby she had lost, even though she never saw or held him. This experience increased the tragedy, as unlike the opportunities we have today, she did not have the ability to see, hold or cuddle her baby or show him that he was loved and would never be forgotten.

## Registration of death and funerals

Many, many years ago the common practice for the burial of stillborn babies was to place them at the foot of another grave, which was done free of charge. Although the parents were told the number of the plot of land, the baby's last resting place remained unmarked. It was also the usual practice for hospitals to offer to dispose of all babies under 28 weeks of gestation (as stillbirth was then only defined by 28 weeks or over), unless the parents wished them to have a private funeral and burial. Private funerals for those babies required the purchase of a plot of land and the family had to bear the cost of the funeral and burial.

Today the interment of all lost babies is treated more humanely, and many local cemeteries have a baby garden where they can be buried, or their ashes scattered free of charge. Hospitals can still provide burials or cremations if the parents wish, and babies can be buried in the same baby garden, or their ashes scattered on it in the usual way, with no involved cost. However, hospitals do not provide individual funerals and the interments only take place when a small group has accumulated.

Parents wishing to have an individual funeral can instruct a local undertaker, who may provide their services free of charge, or at a very reduced rate. If the parents wish, the baby can either be cremated and their ashes scattered on the baby garden, or individually buried and marked with a memorial stone. The same situation applies for babies who have not survived for 24 weeks. I recently became aware of a family who had a funeral with their local undertaker and a burial for their baby lost to miscarriage at only eight weeks of pregnancy. In addition, bereavement midwives from the Trust try to attend the funeral of all lost babies, as a sign of respect and recognition of the family's loss. This all shows the extent to which all human life is now valued and respected, irrespective of how brief the life has been.

At the present time a midwife must complete a birth notification for every baby born alive, even if it is born before 24 completed weeks of pregnancy. If the baby dies after birth, both a live birth and a death have to be registered, which can be done at the same time. A certificate of death is required from the doctor attending the baby. If a baby dies before birth but after 24 completed weeks of pregnancy, this is legally termed a stillbirth. The definition of this, from the Births and Deaths Registration Act 1953, as amended by the Stillbirth Definition Act 1992, is, 'Any child expelled or issued forth from its mother after the 24th week of pregnancy that did not breathe or show any other signs of life.' A certificate is then required to register the death. A midwife who was present at the birth, or who has examined the body afterwards, can issue this certificate and the midwife's signature remains acceptable for registration purposes. However, in practice it is normally a doctor who issues it. After the certificate has been given to the Registrar of births, deaths and marriages, details are entered on a stillbirth register, which is separate register from that of normal births and deaths. A Certificate of Stillbirth is then issued for the baby's burial or cremation.

However, if the baby is born dead after the 24th completed week of pregnancy, but there is medical evidence to indicate that he or she died before 24 weeks, in law this cannot be classed as a stillbirth, and it does not need to be registered as such. Similarly, all babies born dead before 24 weeks are not legally defined as a stillbirth and do not need to be registered. However, society has realized that these babies are potential human beings and they are entitled to the same respect and value we attribute to other human beings. In recognition of this, the RCM recommended in 2008 that hospital Trusts should develop their own hospital-based commemorative Life Certificates for those who have been born too early to be termed stillbirths. The RCM suggested that this could be similar to a generic certificate that had previously been developed by Sands (Sands, 2007). Such a certificate would be useful to show to funeral directors in support of burial or cremation but, more importantly for the family, it would serve to mark the short life of their baby.

If the cause of death of a baby born after 24 weeks is uncertain, the parents may be asked to consent to a hospital post mortem to try to discover this. Parents can refuse permission for this. At present Coroners cannot order a post mortem on a still born child unless there is doubt the child may have been born alive. However, this may change in the future and, if it does, Coroners could have a duty to investigate all stillbirths after 38 weeks gestation.

Over the years the role of midwives involved in stillbirth and neonatal death has gradually evolved and as a result there has been a vast improvement in the type of support given to a mother and her family after such a loss. The development and growth of charities such as Sands has encouraged a change in the way society now views and treats the loss of a baby, even a baby lost to miscarriage at an early gestation. The respect and value we now give indicates an increasing understanding, empathy and compassion for all those who have lost a baby.

However, in the authors' experience, we know that there are still improvements to be made, as even very recently we have heard the accounts of women and their partners who have not received the care and support they deserve. Such experiences surely teach us that there is a great deal yet to be achieved in the training and education of professionals and the more general improvement of services that are, arguably, underfunded. In the future there is also the hope that research will find more ways to prevent the loss of babies who would otherwise never have the chance to live. In the meantime supporting affected families remains a fundamentally important aspect of the midwife's role.

# 9

# Legal issues and overview of the national UK picture

## Legal issues

The current definitions of stillbirth and perinatal death are to be found in the Births and Deaths Registration Act of 1953. Section 41 of that Act defines stillbirth as: 'A child which is issued forth from his mother after 24 weeks of pregnancy and which did not at any time before being completely expelled from its mother breathe or show any other signs of life.'

Following clarifications by the UK Chief Coroner (2023), coroners do not have the jurisdiction to investigate a stillborn child where there has not been an independent life because there has, legally, not been a death. Coroners are able to investigate in the case of a child who is born showing signs of life, whether that is prior to the 24th week of pregnancy or after – even in the case of the mother's pregnancy being intentionally terminated. The guidance goes on to say: 'Where there is doubt over whether a child has been born alive, that is a matter for the coroner to determine.'

Therefore, under the current legal framework, coroners – who are of course independent of health services – are unable to investigate the circumstances surrounding the birth of a stillborn child where there is no evidence of any independent life. As a result, as many have pointed out, families are denied independent investigation. In cases of stillbirth, as well as in cases where the standard of practice of the health professionals involved is below a reasonable standard, it is impossible to learn lessons and, therefore, provide benefit to other professionals working in similar circumstances.

Although internal investigations are carried out by the hospitals where the stillbirth took place, these investigations are rarely independent and, for obvious reasons, our experience of such investigations demonstrates the way in which reports are written in very cautious terms. The only recourse for parents when they are concerned about the standard of care provided is to go to a solicitor and start legal action. Such actions are usually very complicated and it may take months, or years, before there is any end to legal proceedings.

## The facts

Sadly, the loss of a baby is not a very rare experience, as figures from the Office for National Statistics in 2021 have reported. In the UK more than 3,600 stillbirths occur every year; that is, approximately 1 in every 250 births end in a stillbirth. This regrettably means that 8 babies are stillborn every year in the UK (NHS, 2023).

We realize that although some readers will want to know more about the statistics mentioned above and information about causation, some will decide that they want to skip this section and move on to Part 3 of this book, 'Coping and restoration'.

## MBRRACE-UK

The UK is fortunate in having a body that provides an overview of this sad topic. MBRRACE-UK (Mothers and Babies: Reducing Risk through Audits and Confidential Enquiries across the UK) is a collaborative effort that runs alongside the national programme of work conducting surveillance and investigating the causes of maternal deaths, stillbirths and infant deaths.

A report published by MBRRACE-UK in 2016 (MBRRACE-UK, 2023a) stated that for the year 2021 the stillbirth rate (deaths on or after the 24th week of pregnancy) was 3.54 for every 1,000 births. This is probably much higher than the public realize, as a family experiencing the stillbirth may feel that they are the only people who have suffered this tragic event. The report also described the rate of neonatal deaths, which was 1.65 for every 1,000 live births. This rate is split into early neonatal deaths, which includes babies born after 20 weeks of pregnancy weighing 400 g (14 oz) or more who die within seven days of birth, and late neonatal deaths, which refers to those babies dying after seven days but before 28 days.

The combined stillbirth and total neonatal death rates are termed the 'perinatal death rate'. The MBRRACE-UK report stated that the perinatal rate in the UK was higher than those of the best-performing European countries. This may be surprising, given that care is freely available for all in the UK under the NHS.

The MBBRACE-UK report highlighted that women living in the most socially deprived areas of the UK were 50 per cent more likely to have a stillbirth or a neonatal death. In addition, it reported that babies from black, black British or Asian ethnicity had the highest perinatal death rate of all. There are now two specific reports that deal with black and Asian populations; both reports (2023b, 2023c) making recommendations that may serve to reduce stillbirth and early baby loss. It should also be noted that the latest available figures may reflect the situation that prevailed in the UK during the Covid-19 pandemic, although there is no clear association between the pandemic and the cause of early baby loss.

According to the MBBRACE-UK report, however, care should be taken when interpreting the data from areas where mortality rates were higher, as the higher rates may involve more complicated issues. For example, the report recognized that small hospitals with fewer births might have slightly fluctuating numbers of perinatal deaths from year to year, which might give an impression that their rates were rising. In addition, some hospitals provide care for more women in a high-risk category due to the area in which they live, which has greater socioeconomic deprivation. Similarly, the hospital might care for more women with existing medical complications, which involves a greater risk of higher perinatal mortality rate. Therefore, the population mix can influence the geographical appearance of perinatal mortality rates, even if the hospitals in these areas provide high-quality care.

Although not stated in the report, hospitals acting as regional neonatal care centres also have higher neonatal mortality rates, because they receive transfers from elsewhere. These will include the most pre-term or sick babies who might have little chance of survival. It will also include babies delivered following their mothers' transfer in very pre-term labour, when their local hospital could not provide the high level of intensive care the baby would require at birth and afterwards.

The recommendations of the MBBRACE-UK report (2023) include the need to support external clinical input into the vigorous review of all stillbirths and neonatal deaths across the UK. The purpose of external clinical input and the rigorous review that would follow is aimed at identifying the learning and common themes relating to clinical care and service provision, delivery and organization. Other recommendations include the need to improve pathology services so as to identify cause of death, noting that a third of all stillbirths have no cause of death identified. These recommendations follow on from other investigations (for example, the Report of the Morecambe Bay Investigation (Kirkup, 2013)).

To these ends, MBRRACE-UK developed a Perinatal Mortality Reporting Tool in 2018. The Perinatal Mortality Tool is now produced online by the National Perinatal Epidemiology Unit (NPEU, 2018). This allows all hospitals to benefit from lessons learned from others, allowing them to make changes that might reduce perinatal mortality rate. It is worthy of note that the tool has been designed with user and parent involvement.

## Causes of stillbirth and neonatal death

There are a number of maternal conditions that are particularly linked with stillbirth and neonatal death; many of these involve the placenta (the organ that develops in the womb and provides oxygen and nutrients to the baby, at the same time as removing waste products). The placenta is connected to the baby via the umbilical cord.

It is known that the placenta does not function in the best way when the mother has certain medical conditions, including diabetes and high blood pressure, leading to pre-eclampsia. These conditions require extra monitoring during pregnancy and, in the case of diabetes, it is important to ensure that blood sugar levels are kept as normal as possible. Pre-eclampsia may lead to a condition a known as eclampsia, which results in seizures. Sometimes high blood pressure during pregnancy develops gradually but, in other cases, pre-eclampsia can occur without a great deal of warning.

Pre-eclampsia may cause an impairment in the functioning of the placenta; this, in turn, affects the baby in the womb.

Sadly, we know that the use of drugs, alcohol and tobacco during pregnancy is linked to stillbirth and that the babies of women who used drugs, alcohol or tobacco in pregnancy are at greater risk of developmental problems.

Sometimes stillbirth is caused by the placenta becoming detached from the womb; on occasion this is very sudden and places the baby at great risk. It is also well known that there are a range of problems involved with the umbilical cord that can lead to the death of a baby or severe brain damage. With good midwifery and obstetric care, most of the cord problems can be resolved, possibly by undertaking a caesarean section operation.

We also know that maternal infections can lead to stillbirth. There is a range of viral and bacterial conditions that can cause stillbirth, premature birth, low birthweight, or death in the first week of life. If these infections are detected, interventions may be put in place to reduce the risks to both mother and baby.

Even when the cause of stillbirth is known, this does not necessarily mean that there was an intervention that could have prevented it. We live in a day and age where the general public increasingly believes that there is a treatment for all conditions. Sadly, when one looks objectively at the possible causes of stillbirth, it becomes clear that even when a condition is detected during pregnancy, a stillbirth or death shortly after birth cannot be prevented. This can leave parents with a sense of failure if things go wrong, and this may add to their grief. When things go wrong without it being anybody's fault, parents need to be made aware of this so that they are not left feeling guilty, as this would be unjust and leave them with a burden that was very heavy to bear.

However, both authors, who have acted as expert witnesses in many such cases, can say that they have never found a legal claim that was instigated by parents out of a desire for compensation; rather claims were instigated to obtain justice and a desire to prevent the same tragedy happening to other families.

Sadly, lessons are not easily learned, as we often see the same mistakes happening over and over again, which leaves us with a sense of deep sadness and regret. The process of obtaining compensation, however, is by way of an adversarial system that can be arduous, with the outcome unsure. Not all parents are willing to go through what is a painful and stressful process. It is questionable whether gaining the knowledge that somebody was to blame for the loss of a baby can make it easier for parents to bear, or whether the alternative is true – that it was worse to think somebody caused the death of their child. However, even when legal claims are successful there are no winners, which is something that we professionals should remember.

A consideration of the causes of stillbirth leads one to the conclusion that regular monitoring of the pregnancy by midwives and the use of scans and blood tests is essential for all mothers to be, especially for those at risk. As the rates of stillbirth in the UK are higher than those in other European countries, there is clearly considerable room for improvement.

# Part 3
# COPING AND RESTORATION

## Introduction to Part 3

Throughout Part 3 of this book there will be many references to cognitive behavioural therapy (CBT). CBT is now, perhaps, the most widely available therapy and there is a great deal of evidence to show that it is a very successful treatment. This is not to say that CBT is a panacea and, indeed, there is evidence that other forms of treatment without medication (for example, some of the psychotherapies and counselling) may be very helpful. Among the psychotherapies, CBT is probably unique insofar as there is now a wide range of resources – books, apps and online programmes – that individuals may use as self-help, without the need to access a health professional. The NHS website (<www.nhs.uk>) has an excellent section on CBT, which describes how it works, the conditions for which it is helpful and what happens during professionally developed sessions.

One of the best definitions of CBT comes from Dr Judith Beck, of the Beck Institute, Pennsylvania, USA. She says (Beck, 2011):

> CBT is one of the few forms of psychotherapy that has been scientifically tested and found to be effective in hundreds of clinical trials, for many different disorders. In contrast to other forms of psychotherapy, CBT is usually more focused on the present, more time-limited, and more problem-solving oriented. In addition, patients learn special skills that they can use for the rest of their lives. These skills involve identifying distorted thinking, modifying beliefs, relating to others in different ways, and changing behaviours.

Therefore, CBT doesn't involve 'analysing' you; it doesn't subscribe to the theories of Freud and Jung; and your therapist doesn't ask you to lie on a couch while she/he discusses your unconscious.

In the process of therapy your therapist will work with you and find ways that you can help yourself.

One of the most common presentations of women who have experienced stillbirth or new baby death is that of profound feelings of grief together with PTSD or many of the features of PTSD. The central components of CBT for PTSD include:

- helping the person face up to memories of the traumatic event, including helping them to imagine the event and relive it in the present tense, including all the thoughts and feelings associated with it;
- exposure to situations that evoke memories – in particular and where possible, helping the person visit the scene where the event took place;
- providing the person with education about the nature of PTSD and, in particular, identifying factors known to increase difficulties, such as the use of drugs and alcohol, avoidance behaviour and so on;
- general anxiety-management training;
- engaging members of the family and/or significant others to help with rehabilitation;
- dealing with any associated abuse of drugs and/or alcohol;
- developing coping strategies.

CBT is now widely available in the UK in an NHS programme (NHS Talking Therapies for Anxiety and Depression). This programme was formerly known as the Improving Access to Psychological Therapies (IAPT) programme. Since the programme was developed, over a decade ago, more than one million people have benefitted from treatment. The title of the programme is somewhat misleading as, in addition to states of anxiety and depression, the programme offers treatment for a number of other conditions, including health anxiety, obsessive compulsive disorder and post-traumatic stress disorder. Therefore, this programme is invaluable to many of those who have suffered stillbirth and early baby loss.

The NHS Talking Therapies Programme employs both a 'low-intensity' and a 'high-intensity' approach to people's problems. This is based on the principle that one should start with the simple interventions ('low intensity'), such as self-help and guided reading. Only when such methods have not been effective, should one move to the next step (perhaps a short course of therapy from a nurse practitioner or a low intensity therapist). Thereafter, if necessary, one may move to ('high-intensity') therapy from a clinical psychologist, or specially trained nurse therapist and then to more complex interventions; these may include specialist CBT, with or without a combination of medication.

# 10

## Coping with the loss

Some women and their partners will, eventually, without any help or advice, deal with their loss in their own way. Over time they will develop coping mechanisms that, eventually, restore them to a reasonable level of function and the ability to enjoy life once more. The research literature tells us something of this process, and that a significant proportion of people will, if left to their own devices, cope with their loss and are restored to 'normality'. However, the research literature tells us nothing about how long these processes take. It has been our experience that some women and their partners can achieve a return to 'normality' within weeks, or a couple of months. For others that process may last many months. However, that is not to say that their sense of loss disappears.

Some people will need to receive professional treatment (for example, for particular symptoms that might be seen in a depressive illness, or PTSD). However, the research literature makes it clear that there is no single professional intervention that will lead to a resolution of the psychological and emotional distress that follows a stillbirth. *The Lancet* review, mentioned in Chapter 1, helpfully summarizes their extensive review of the published literature of research studies conducted in a number of countries. For anyone interested in reading this report, we recommend reading the original paper, which is, very helpfully, relatively free from jargon, and therefore reasonably easy to read and digest (*The Lancet*, 2016).

As we have indicated earlier, it has been our experience that it is impossible to generalize about the effects of stillbirth on individuals, as every case is unique. Some people are affected in certain ways, other not. With regard to what works, there is plentiful evidence of a considerable variation in the way that individuals respond to self-help, attendance at support groups, treatments delivered by professionals (for example, CBT or medication), or indeed, as noted above, simply allowing time for the process of natural healing to take place. Some people respond to a specific intervention and obtain very substantial benefits; others obtain only minor benefits or, in some cases, the interventions that are offered are unacceptable to that particular individual (for a whole range of reasons).

Before describing self-help and professional interventions, it is, in our opinion, important to emphasize that other, more general factors come into play in helping affected people. It appears to us that there are three particular components of importance in addition to treatments and self-help. These are:

- the role of the family and friends;
- support groups;
- employment and other activities.

## The role of the family and friends

In general, families and friends rally around in the aftermath of the tragedy of stillbirth and perinatal death. The woman and her partner often receive a great deal of attention and care. However, for most of us who have contact with someone who has gone through such a bereavement (or indeed any bereavement), life simply goes on and we tend to forget that those affected might continue to suffer and continue to need our support. When life goes on we become preoccupied by events in the present, problems or happy events in our own lives. Therefore the support that we have previously provided to the affected individuals will tail off. To compound matters, those affected by the tragedy will, in many cases, shut themselves off from contact with the outside world, thus depriving themselves of access to support and comfort.

Our advice to affected individuals is to be as open as possible with your family and friends about what you might need and how you are feeling. Unless they are told they may well assume that all is well. Some family members and friends sometimes have great difficulty in asking 'How are you?' because it is often so difficult for them to know whether they are doing the right thing. It may be that the question, 'How are you?' will cause upset.

Our advice to affected individuals is to be aware that you need to reach out, although it may seem very difficult to keep in touch with friends and not neglect those relationships. It seems clear from our experience that those with supportive families and friends who are aware of the emotional and psychological suffering do much better in the longer term than those who remain isolated. Remember that human interaction is a two-way process and that you will need to make the effort to reach out.

In this section we also need to include the comfort and support that those with a religious faith may obtain through religious rituals and the support of a priest, pastor, rabbi or imam. These individuals have a great deal of experience in helping people through difficult emotional times and one should not be reluctant to ask them for their help. In a sense it is also their 'duty' to do what they can for their parishioners or followers.

## Support groups

In this book we have mentioned the work of support groups, in particular that of Sands. This is not in any way meant to minimize the positive effect of other organizations; this emphasis is solely due to our very positive experience of Sands over many years, and the enormous influence it has in this area.

Support groups principally provide comfort by allowing individuals to meet others who have been through a similar loss. We know that the first encounters with others can be off-putting because of the way in which one's emotions may be triggered or, sometimes, because it is difficult to tolerate the distress that one might see in other affected individuals. However, we know that most people who attend support groups, if they persist, will be provided with invaluable short- and long-term support, practical assistance with coping with symptoms and advice about a range of matters. In our experience, these groups often help people on the journey back to a resumption of normal activities – a reduction in normal activities is, sadly, one of the common consequences of loss.

## Employment and other activities

We know from our experience, and from the research that has been carried out, that being supported and assisted by a sympathetic employer has enormous benefits. Many employers now recognize that going back to work, for either a woman or her partner, represents a huge challenge. Following an occupation you enjoy provides obvious benefits. However, not all individuals are blessed with doing a job they really enjoy. Nevertheless, even for those whose 'job is just a job' one of the obvious benefits is that of distraction from one's thinking. In turn, going to work demands the adoption a normal work-day routine and increases a person's general level of activity and engagement with others.

For many women and their partners, one of the biggest challenges in going back to work is facing their work colleagues. Sometimes, work colleagues just don't know what to say, or how to say it. Many avoid the topic of the loss. In our experience this makes going back to work very difficult. One common problem that arises is the fear that going back to work might involve seeing pregnant women, or women who have recently given birth to a healthy baby. In some occupations one might come across others who have not heard about the loss and may ask such questions as, 'How's life, with an addition to the family?'

There is no easy way to confront these problems. However, employers may assist – as, to their credit, many do – by agreeing on a 'phased return to work schedule'. Some employers agree to a schedule of return to work over many weeks, perhaps beginning with a few hours two days a week, and then gradually building up. The majority of the larger employers will have sympathetic human resource departments and occupational health advisers. In smaller companies and businesses, a phased return to work is not always easily managed and, therefore, going back to work may represent a great challenge.

There are two important pieces of advice that we should give at this point. The first is not to respond to an immediate inclination to resign from one's job. This happens usually because the individual concerned simply cannot face a return to work, in that particular environment, at that time. One needs to allow oneself sufficient time to come to a balanced decision about what is best. It is certainly true that a change of jobs – carrying out the same duties, but in a different setting – may be advisable. However, once more, we would say that a person should not make a major decision like this without giving things sufficient time before acting.

The second piece of advice is not to return to work too soon. One needs time to recover from the traumatic event. While it is obviously important to regain normal activities, returning to work too soon may lead to a range of problems. For example, throwing oneself into work may prevent one from going through a 'normal' process of grieving. It has also been our experience that some individuals throw themselves into work to the extent that nothing else matters. This situation often causes enormous problems in relationships and, sometimes, although the individual may spend many hours at work, their underlying distress may serve to reduce the quality of the work that they do.

# 11

# Self-help – practical measures

Self-help needs to start with addressing some of the basics in life. Although what follows is aimed at assisting those who have suffered loss, our advice also applies to many other people facing different situations. The topics in this section are as follows.

- Talk about it!
- Improve your sleep
- Work on becoming calm – mindfulness, relaxation, breathing exercises
- Exercise
- Improve your diet.

## Talk about it!

Whatever trauma one has suffered, including stillbirth or perinatal death, there is a need to 'talk about it'. However, this is not easy and, sometimes, talking may need to be done with a professional, rather than a family member or friend. In selecting the person that you talk to, you have to remember that some people will 'never get it' and may give very upsetting advice, for example: 'You just need to have another baby.' Sadly, it has been our experience that, in the past (but hopefully not now), this advice has been offered by GPs and other health professionals.

It is also important to talk to someone who will respect your confidentiality and also to remember that the kind and sensitive people who may come to mind when you think about 'talking about it' may become so upset at what you say that they simply cannot cope.

In the early days after stillbirth or perinatal death, professionals tend to offer their time and be very sympathetic to one's upset. However, as time goes by, busy GPs will often simply treat the event as 'water under the bridge', particularly if you show outwardly, as many people do, a calm and reasonably happy demeanour. However, at the same time you may be experiencing a great deal of suffering inside. It is therefore important that, if weeks and months have elapsed and you still have very strong, distressing feelings, you need to reach out to others.

Here it is worth mentioning the role of the health visitors. Health visitors are Registered Nurses who have undergone specialist training. Health visitors, as their name suggests, fulfil their role in the community, by visiting family homes and by giving advice and support to all age groups. However, they have a particular focus on children and families. Health visitors are required to perform statutory checks at 28 weeks of pregnancy, at 10–14 days after birth and at three points thereafter, until the baby reaches two years of age. In the case of stillbirth, health visitors may provide the mother with aftercare. Indeed, the health visitor's role in recognizing and managing mental health problems is now widely recognized.

## What can I do if I can't talk about it?

If you cannot talk about your feelings, one strategy that may be helpful is to write down your story. Our advice is to do this in stages. Write down one account, then look at this and fill in the detail. Leave the account for a day or two, read what you have written, and then start all over again. Keep this process going, filling in details as you go. You will probably find this upsetting, so take your time. Leave it for a while if it causes you to get too upset – but keep at it!

Most people these days like to use a computer, a tablet or similar device for writing their story, particularly because these make editing easier. However, there's nothing wrong with good old-fashioned pen and paper. Some people benefit from describing their story in picture form – in sketches, or in paintings. It doesn't matter if you're not a world-class artist: if you think drawing or painting will be helpful, then do it! Expressing your feelings is the priority. Sometimes people benefit from making recordings. These can be made on your smartphone, on a dictaphone or by video.

The experience of putting together one's story on paper, or on a computer, in pictures and drawings or, in some cases, in poetry can be therapeutic in itself. However, it is usually helpful to share what you have produced with another person. In the course of professional treatment the therapist may ask individuals to provide a written account and thereafter to keep a diary of their thoughts, feelings and mood as well as telling the therapist during the treatment sessions.

## Improve your sleep

Sleeping problems are a common consequence of loss. Some find sleep comes very quickly, but then they wake very early in the morning (at 3 or 4 o'clock). Conversely, others find they can't get to sleep for several hours, and toss and turn, but eventually sleep for only a few hours before waking. Others report sleep of poor quality, when they might be in bed and asleep for a reasonable period of time, but will be aware of being restless and having frequent dreams or nightmares. For some sleep is an escape. It is not unusual to see those who, quite literally, hide under the covers. Excessive sleep may worsen mood and perversely may reduce energy levels.

All of these sleep problems lead to feeling tired and unrefreshed in the morning. Sleep and the reasons why we sleep are still, in many ways, life mysteries. However, we know that sleep is a vital factor in contributing to good health and well-being. While sleep problems may obviously be caused by loss, there are many ways in which you can at least improve your sleep. This is important because poor sleep may lead to a range of problems, including an increased risk of type 2 diabetes, a risk of putting on excess weight and an overall reduction in sharpness of thinking.

How, then, might sleep be improved? Keeping to a routine is really important. Begin with setting an alarm to wake every morning at the same time and only going to bed when you are sleepy. If you wake in the night, don't stay in bed and 'toss and turn' – if after a few minutes you are still not falling back to sleep, get up, leave the bedroom and go and do something that does not stimulate you, such as doing a crossword, doing some sewing or playing patience. When you are a little more relaxed and the thoughts that have kept you awake recede, you can try going back to bed.

One of the most important modern-day causes of sleep disturbance is the environment that we have created for ourselves, that is, bedrooms with televisions and iPads, Kindles and telephones on our bedside tables. There is now a growing body of research suggesting that, in the period leading up to bedtime, it is advisable to ban the use of all devices because of the glow that these produce. The light from our electronic devices serves to fool our brains into believing that it is 'stay awake' time rather than 'go to sleep' time. It has been pointed out that the electronic devices emit the same wavelength of light as sunshine.

For many of us, having a ban on electronic devices is difficult to contemplate, and many will say that they need to keep up to date with Facebook postings, Instagram, Twitter (hearing the latest opinions on current events), email, text messages, WhatsApp and so on. Unless you are the police commander on call for major incidents, or have a similar, demanding role, it is difficult, when one thinks about it, to understand why messages and postings cannot wait until the next day. Unfortunately, our culture has reinforced the view that our phones and computers need to be permanently turned on. Apart from the damage to sleep, it is becoming increasingly obvious that our addiction to electronic devices may cause more widespread problems, not least the reduction of face-to-face human interaction.

Having a television in the bedroom is, in our opinion, a great mistake. Bedrooms are for sleeping, not for keeping up with the news or the latest streaming from one of the online platforms. By all means, watch a film that finishes half an hour or so before you go to bed; this may actually enhance a feeling of well-being, particularly if it is light-hearted and humorous, rather than terrifying or gory.

There are also some simple measures that one can take in the bedroom to enhance sleep. There is plentiful consumer research that shows we pay little attention to our beds and mattresses, and many of us sleep on mattresses that are many years beyond their 'use by' dates. Similarly, with pillows, having a good pillow is not a luxury, but a necessity. Spending a few more pounds on the most comfortable pillows and changing them on a reasonably regular basis may produce untold benefits.

It is also advisable to make your room one of absolute darkness. To do this you might have to think about putting heavy curtains in place. It is also advisable, most times of the year, to let some air in, although this may be impossible if you live on a busy road. Sometimes one needs to weigh the benefit of fresh air against the occasional noise from a passing car or birdsong. We do realize, however, that not all of us can live in houses deep in the countryside! You might consider opening the bedroom windows wide in the hours leading up to bedtime, to make the room as cool as possible. Fortunately for those readers in the UK, heat at night is relatively rare. One other useful piece of advice on warm nights is to take a warm, rather than a cool shower. A cool shower reduces skin temperature and tells the brain to warm up the body, thus making a warm night even warmer.

Another important factor in setting a sleep routine is to try to get outside in the daylight as soon as possible after waking. A 10- to 15-minute walk (even if you have to set your alarm 10–15 minutes early) will yield untold benefits. The exposure to light in the morning helps to reset your body clock.

## Work on becoming calm

As with exercise, which we will discuss below, people who have experienced loss will not have relaxation at the top of their agenda. However, experience has taught us that acquiring skills that reduce physical tension and mental preoccupation is an essential part of coping and resolution.

To begin, you need to set aside time for yourself. This might be just ten minutes during the day to put your feet up and read your Kindle or to walk to the nearest café and have a tea or coffee. Some find listening to music relaxing. Activities such as these are not the first to come to mind if you are preoccupied by loss.

There are many ways that one can reduce physical tension and empty one's mind of distressing thoughts. Experience has taught us that there is no single strategy that works best, and that one needs to bear in mind the considerable individual differences that occur across the human race. There are well-proven strategies such as mindfulness (more of that below) that help many achieve relaxation.

However, some people simply prefer to relax by spending time, for example, sketching, painting or joining one of the community choirs that are proliferating across the country.

There are, of course, enormous benefits to joining a community activity such as a choir. The majority of choirs will take people at all levels of ability, without the need for an audition or to pass any kind of test. Community choirs consist of people from all walks of life and ages (and shapes and sizes!). The words of a song may be relaxing in themselves. Singing also has enormous benefits in respect of muscle relaxation, due to the breathing control that one learns over time. Such choirs yield other benefits, including distraction and perhaps the development of long-term friendships, apart, that is, from the pure joy that music brings to many. (To find a choir, try <http://www.bbc.co.uk/sing/findachoir.shtml>.)

## Mindfulness

Mindfulness is a form of meditation and is now used widely across the NHS as a formal treatment. Its use is supported by an evidence base that shows it is effective for a number of mental health problems. In our opinion it is particularly useful for those who have suffered loss and need to deal with intrusive and distressing memories or who, at times, become preoccupied by particular distressing thoughts.

So, what is mindfulness? The approach is, in essence, simple. A generally accepted definition reads as follows: The intentional accepting and non-judgemental focusing of on one's attention on the emotions, thoughts and sensations of being in the present moment. There are many mindfulness techniques, which may simply involve a focus on breathing or on aspects of your environment. The techniques take some time to learn and practise. Research evidence shows that mindfulness and other meditation techniques lower blood pressure and improve sleep and concentration. There is also research that shows (using sophisticated scanning technology) that mindfulness alters (for the better) brain function (MAPPG, 2015).

Mindfulness has now become an industry and there are many commercial organizations marketing mindfulness courses, some of these at quite considerable expense. An alternative is to visit the website of the Mental Health Foundation, a leading UK mental health charity, and look for further information about mindfulness. The Mental Health Foundation markets an online course for a small charge (see <www.mentalhealth.org.uk/a-to-z/m/mindfulness>). The course can be taken in your own time and on your phone, tablet or PC.

An NHS review of mindfulness can be found at <https://themindfulnessinitiative.org.uk/images/reports/Mindfulness-APPG-Report_Mindful-Nation-UK_Oct2015.pdf>.

## Relaxation

Mindfulness is but one way to obtain relaxation and acquire the skill to focus on thoughts that do not cause distress. Simple relaxation techniques have been long used to obtain physical and mental relaxation. Progressive muscle relaxation training uses a focus on systematically tensing and relaxing the muscles of the body. It helps you to differentiate between states of tension and relaxation and, importantly, recognize when your level of muscle tension is increasing.

Many people who are anxious do not realize just how physically tense they are, this tension being evident as headaches, neck stiffness and other physical symptoms. The recognition of muscle tension is important and, in the exercises that involve tensing your muscles voluntarily, you begin to realize once tension is released just what relaxation feels like. There is considerable evidence to suggest that systematic tensing and relaxing exercises eventually lead to a state of overall muscle relaxation and, as a consequence, a feeling of well-being.

The following exercise is straightforward. It may be helpful to read and inwardly digest the instructions and then make a recording of your own voice that you can follow. However, there are also many commercially available exercises or some freely available at the click of a button on a website. One such example can be found at <https://www.helpguide.org/articles/stress/relaxation-techniques-for-stress-relief.htm/>.

Muscle relaxation exercises combat the body's fight or flight response, which is produced in states of anxiety, depression, emotional distress and PTSD. In the emotional numbness that one may feel after trauma, the nervous system – in a sense – becomes 'stuck' and one feels numb and frozen. In such states muscle relaxation may be a helpful antidote.

### Try this

Before doing the exercises it is important to remember that tensing your muscles should be done to a moderate extent. If you tense them too hard, you will defeat the object of the exercise. A simple guide is that tensing of muscles should lead to no more than a sensation of tensing or 'pulling'. If you experience pain, you are trying too hard. Further, when you release the tension, you should feel it go immediately.

Plan in advance, so identify a time in the day when you have 30 minutes to devote to this task. Find a quiet room, turn off your mobile, unplug the landline and wear loose, comfortable clothing. The exercise can be carried out in a comfortable chair or lying down, and you should experiment with different situations and times of the day to identify what the optimum conditions are for you.

---

### Deep muscle relaxation exercise

- Get in position and begin with your right hand. Clench your fist so that your knuckles are white. Hold for 5 seconds, then release immediately.
- Pause, wait 10 seconds, and then repeat.
- Tense your right forearm, closing your fist and tensing the muscles of your forearm. Remember: not too hard. Hold for 5 seconds, then release immediately.
- Pause, wait 10 seconds, and then repeat.
- Tense your right biceps by clenching your fist and bending your arm, so that it forms a 90 degree angle. Concentrate on making your biceps bulge as much as possible. Hold for 5 seconds, then release immediately.
- Pause, wait 10 seconds, and then repeat.
- Repeat these actions with the left hand, forearm and biceps. Remembering to do each exercise twice, hold for 5 seconds, and then release immediately.
- Next move your head and neck. Tense your eye muscles by screwing them up. Keep your eyes and keep them shut tight. Hold for and seconds, and then release immediately.

- Pause, wait 10 seconds, and then repeat.
- Tense your mouth by clenching your jaws together, and concentrate on pressing your lips together as firmly as possible. At the same time you will notice that you tense your eyes. Hold for 5 seconds, then release immediately.
- Pause, wait 10 seconds, and then repeat.
- Now concentrate on tensing your neck. Push your chin down a little towards your chest but do not let it touch your chest. Hold for 5 seconds, then release immediately.
- Pause, wait 10 seconds, and then repeat.
- Next, move your shoulders and back, pushing your shoulders up slightly and tensing your neck. Feel the muscles tighten across your shoulders. Hold for 5 seconds, then release immediately.
- Pause, wait 10 seconds, and then repeat.
- Tense your shoulders and arms by pushing your arms down, holding your neck rigid. Concentrate on tensing across your shoulders. Hold for 5 seconds, then release immediately.
- Pause, wait 10 seconds, and then repeat.
- Tense the muscles in your back by pushing your elbows into your sides, pulling your shoulders down, holding your neck tight and pushing your head down towards your chest, concentrating on tensing the muscles across your back. Hold for 5 seconds, then release immediately.
- Pause, wait 10 seconds, and then repeat.
- Now move to your chest and abdomen. Tense the muscles of your chest by pushing your shoulders back, pushing your elbows down into your waist and tilting your head back slightly, concentrating on holding your chest in a barrel-like, rigid way. Hold for 5 seconds, then release immediately.
- Pause, wait 10 seconds, and then repeat.
- Tense the muscles of your stomach from the back and pull in towards your navel. Hold for 5 seconds, then release immediately.
- Pause, wait 10 seconds, and then repeat.
- Next, move to your lower body and legs. Tense your thighs and buttocks by pushing your buttocks down, and concentrate on tensing your thighs and buttocks together. Hold for 5 seconds, then release immediately.
- Pause, wait 10 seconds, and then repeat.
- Tense your right calf by pulling your toes up towards you, keeping your leg straight at the knee. Pull your toes back until

you can feel the pull all the way up your calf muscles. Hold for 5 seconds, then release immediately.

- Pause, wait 10 seconds, and then repeat.
- Tense your right foot by curling your toes, trying to make them clench like a fist. Hold for 5 seconds, then release immediately.
- Pause, wait 10 seconds, and then repeat.
- Repeat this sequence for your left calf and foot.
- When you come to this point, begin to tense your whole body, starting with your hands, working up through your arms, then your head, neck, shoulders, back, chest, stomach, buttocks, thighs, calves and feet. Take 10 seconds to gradually tense the whole body. Hold for 5 seconds, then relax.
- As you relax breathe out as much as you can, slowly. Keep your eyes closed and say 'calm' to yourself.
- Repeat this last sequence – tensing your whole body and ending by saying 'calm' to yourself – five times, remembering to leave 10 seconds between each.
- Next, concentrate on slowing down your breathing. Try to feel all your chest and, as you breathe out, say 'calm' to yourself. Let your breathing settle into a natural rhythm and then try to fix your mind on a quiet and relaxing scene. Imagine yourself lying on a beach or in a meadow. Imagine a warm atmosphere around you. Try to image the smells of this environment. Keep your mind as fixed on this place as possible and let yourself drift. Don't worry if you fall asleep, but it may be worth setting your alarm clock first!

## Breathing exercises

Breathing exercises can be an effective way of dealing with high levels of anxiety. They can also be helpful at times when you simply need to calm down. Controlling your breathing not only gives you a feeling of calm, but also reduces your blood pressure and generally reduces stress on the body. Remember that relaxed breathing should involve all the chest and diaphragm. Breathing from the top of the chest – the anxious breathing that we all experience at times – promotes more anxiety.

One of the most important things about controlled breathing is to slow down your breathing rate gradually, so that eventually you are breathing 6–8 times a minute, instead of 12, 14, 16 or more.

**Breathing exercise**

- Find somewhere to relax (a nice comfortable chair is better than a bed), and put one hand at the top of your chest and the other on your upper abdomen.
- Breathe in through your nose, making sure the whole chest inflates.
- You can feel this by the movement in your hands. Breathe very slowly in.
- Hold the breath and then exhale slowly.
- Another trick that is often used is alternate-nostril breathing, something often practised in yoga classes.
- Sit for a while in a comfortable chair and relax as much as possible.
- Pace your right thumb over your right nostril and breathe in through your left nostril. When you have taken in a deep breath, close off your left nostril and exhale through your right nostril.
- Continue this breathing for 5–10 minutes

Breathing exercises often work well after you have practised deep-muscle relaxation techniques. A useful app can be found at <www.calm.com/breathe>.

## Exercise

When one is low in mood, perhaps preoccupied by very sombre and depressing thoughts, the last thing that comes to mind is physical exercise. However, exercise is, of course, an essential ingredient in maintaining good health. Perhaps you do not need to be told that a lack of exercise is linked with a greatly increased risk of developing a number of health problems, notably those affecting the heart and circulation, but also other vital systems. Longer term, the weight gain associated with lack of exercise may lead to type 2 diabetes, problems with hips and joints and is, as we know now, linked to an increased risk of dementia in the longer term. For women who have been pregnant, exercise is an essential ingredient in losing weight and toning their body once more. Again, it needs to be said that for a woman who has lost a baby after months of pregnancy, and who is still recovering both physically and emotionally, exercise does not come readily to mind as a preferred activity. Similarly, 'toning one's body' is not seen as a priority.

With regard to the low mood and anxiety so commonly associated with loss, exercise is perhaps one of the best interventions. We now know that for those with mild to moderate levels of depression, exercise is a first-line treatment and is recommended by NICE. It is also clear, from a number of studies, conducted both nationally and internationally, that exercise may be as beneficial for mild to moderate levels of depression as antidepressants and talking therapies such as CBT. Alongside the production of the body's own mood-enhancing chemicals, participation in exercise will also mean an increase in social interaction. Following exercise, and rather counter-intuitively, you may see an increase in energy and motivation towards other activities.

## So what types of exercise are beneficial?

The answer to this is anything that gets you active. Walking when you might drive, gardening and do-it-yourself all keep you active and improve the health of your joints and muscles. That said, the greatest beneficial impact on mood and physical health comes from exercise such as brisk walking, running, swimming or cycling. Simply put, these forms of exercise get our hearts and lungs going and get us slightly out of breath. One simple rule of thumb is that beneficial exercise should involve getting out of breath for reasonably lengthy periods (20 minutes or more three or four times a week), but not so much out of breath that you cannot say a few words, sing a little or hold a simple conversation. Longer periods of exercise may be more beneficial, and becoming physically tired for a while after is not bad thing.

One note of caution, if you have not exercised for a while and have any significant health problems, you need to speak to your GP before starting an exercise programme. Also remember that you will need to approach any exercise with the knowledge that you need to build this up over time – it is important to emphasize 'graduated doses'.

## Parkrun

- To improve motivation, you might think of signing up for 'parkrun' (for more information go to <www.parkrun.org>). Parkrun is a totally free of charge activity held at 9 a.m. every Saturday morning throughout the UK. There are few places where parkrun is not available within a 30-minute drive. Parkruns are, as the word implies, running in parks and open spaces. They consist of a 5-km (just over 3-mile) course.
- At this point, for those non-runners or those who consider themselves grossly out of shape, don't give up reading! When one visits a parkrun, one is struck by the range, size and speed of those taking part. While it is true that the fastest parkrunners will run the 5-km course in 16 minutes or thereabouts, one will also see people with morbid obesity at the same event who complete the course in an hour or more. In between, there is a whole spectrum of fitness and ages. Parkrun is also different from many of the fun runs that are advertised, insofar as the level of competitiveness is just enough to keep people trying to complete the course in a faster time, but not so great that slower runners feel in any way ashamed at their accomplishment. If one routinely goes to the same location, what is impressive is the level of social interaction between people of many diverse backgrounds who, in the normal course of life, would not meet each other.
- Parkruns are simple to sign up for – go to the website, put in a few personal details (name, age and email address) and, once this is complete download the barcode. Just turn up for the event and when you finish you will be handed a wooden chip, which you take along with your barcode to a meeting point. These will be scanned into a computer. Within hours you will be able to see your results on the email automatically sent to you and compare them with age-related averages. One enormous plus for the parkrun is that this is absolutely free. It is supported by a number of charities and also by commercial sponsorship. Across the UK and beyond there are now hundreds of thousands of people completing parkrun every week. Some people also use the parkrun as a way of exploring new places.
- There are now parkrun events for children aged 4–14 years (see <www.parkrun.org.uk/events/juniorevents/>) over a 2-km course, although children are also welcome at the adult version.

There are plenty of 12- and 13-year-olds running around with their parents at the adult version. You will also see people with dogs on short leads and blind runners accompanied by a friend. One note of caution is that, at most parkruns, you will see a man or a woman running with a baby in a buggy. Although this may be upsetting, perhaps this should be regarded as a challenge that one must eventually face in resuming a normal life and existence.

Joining clubs and registering for the gym are other alternatives. Most areas have cycling and netball, as well as walking football and netball for those of lesser initial ability. Contrary to popular belief most athletic clubs will encourage absolute beginners to join and will offer coaching, aimed at getting a person started. Many people we have seen who have experienced loss use events to raise money for good causes. We know many individuals who have set up their own charities in the name of the lost baby or who run, walk or cycle for Sands or similar organizations.

In addition to exercise such as the gym, running and cycling, just increasing your level of activity will be beneficial to mood and health. You might, therefore, consider buying a Fitbit (or similar device) and aim to walk 10,000 steps each day. You will be surprised at just how easy this is to reach by walking instead of taking a car and going for an extra stroll every day. These devices also register your resting heart rate. This is important as resting heart rates fall with increased fitness and one can track progress by observing this. This will therefore motivate you even further. Another benefit is that these devices will record sleep. It is probably a universal truth that people who exercise more sleep better. Finally, don't think that you need to run a marathon or do the London to Brighton cycle ride to your improve health – simple adjustments to your daily routine (taking the stairs instead of using the lift, or walking instead of using the car) will bring benefits.

It is also really important to find a way that suits you to keep your body stretched and toned. One can do this in five to ten minutes at home with some press-ups, squats or lunges – perhaps you could invest in a book with some instructions. Stretching is a great way of preventing stiff backs and necks. For exercise ideas, try the NHS advice 'Get active your way' at <https://www.nhs.uk/live-well/exercise/get-active-your-way/>.

## Improve your diet

There is, of course, massive evidence that many of us do not eat well. For those with any mental health problems, and perhaps more so for those immersed in a grieving process, diet is often neglected, with a reduction in appetite, and simply 'eating to live'. In this section we will not provide comprehensive advice about the matter of diet; rather, we will set out our advice on some of the basics and provide some useful links to those who have a lot more to say on the subject. There are, however, some basics about diet that are particularly applicable to the parents who are the subject of this book. Some of what we have to say is very simple but, nevertheless, we feel that there is a need to repeat some important messages.

First, drink sufficient water. There appears to be a consensus that many of us do not drink enough water. Most authorities suggest that at least two litres per day is the minimum amount, with more if you exercise at any level of intensity. When given this advice many will say that, 'This is too much, I'll be forever going to the loo!' One indicator of drinking sufficient amounts of water is the colour of your urine. This should be a pale, straw colour rather than deeper yellow or orange. On the topic of a reasonable fluid intake, it is also worth mentioning that you might, perhaps, switch to water rather than fizzy drinks. Fizzy drinks often contain either a high calorie content or preservatives, or both. Also try to remember that caffeinated drinks, such as tea, coffee and colas, are diuretics, that is, they all stimulate urination and can lead to dehydration.

So why should you drink more? There are a number of very good reasons for this, notably flushing out the body's toxins and preventing conditions such as kidney stones. Drinking water may actually increase the number of calories that you burn and assist with the digestive process. Not drinking enough leads to dehydration, which, in the early stages, can cause headaches and a 'fogginess' of thinking. Severe dehydration is obviously more serious and causes problems with the balance of salts and electrolytes in your body. If you are constantly dehydrated, even at a mild level, you are very likely to become physically weaker and suffer fatigue.

In our opinion, another important element of diet is the eating of plenty of fruit and vegetables – the so-called five-a-day advice. There is some controversy about the number of portions of fruit and vegetables a day that are necessary to maintain good health, the UK government advising fewer than other countries, which set the guidance at a much higher level. In Australia, the government suggests seven-a-day, Canada up to ten-a-day and Japan even more. In the links we provide below you will find plenty of advice about the types of fruit and vegetables that are best for you.

What about fast food? So often we hear parents say, 'I've given up cooking meals. When I do want to eat, and that's not very often, I'm relying on fast foods and takeaways.' We of course appreciate that, with low levels of motivation, cooking an extravagant meal is the last thing you want to do. However, just remember that it probably takes less effort and is considerably cheaper to have beans on toast, or to put a jacket potato in the microwave.

Our final piece of advice is to ensure that, at least once a day, the family eats together at the table, with a ban on the use of electronic devices. The benefits of this are obvious.

There are two sources of advice on diet that we have found extremely helpful and based on sound scientific evidence.

The first is to be found in a book by GP, author, television presenter and podcaster Dr Rangan Chatterjee. A large section of his book, *The 4 Pillar Plan*, is devoted to diet, with some simple advice conveyed in a very readable form. Dr Chatterjee also expands in three other topics we have mentioned in this chapter: relaxation, movement and sleep.

The second source of information is a blog by psychiatrist and former GP Dr Michael Beary (<mikebeary.blogspot.com>). Michael has been a colleague of one of the authors for more than 30 years. A summary of his advice (derived from his various blog posts) is set out below:

We now have good scientific proof that the right healthy diet not only improves our general health but also improves mental health and reduces our need for treatment from our doctor for conditions such as depression.

Happily this turns out to be pretty much what I have been advocating over many years.

The version of the Mediterranean diet that I advise my patients to follow is to eat 26 different natural foods of many colours including olive oil every day.

This is an easy way to be sure you are eating a Mediterranean diet. Various fish such as mackerel and herring are always a good idea in a salad as are nuts and seeds provided you have no allergies. Muesli is always an option for breakfast and the milk counts as one food. Typically this means you start the day off with 6 or more of your varied foods.

All the many previous research studies over many years have had the potential for bias in favor of the sponsor's product such as a 'health' spread or commercial supplement.

What was needed was a very systematic research programme following patients carefully over a number of years comparing more than one different diet with all the scientific pitfalls covered.

The Spanish PREDIMED study is the only unsponsored, prospective, randomized trial ever conducted worldwide in this field and therefore the only one that can be relied upon scientifically.

Interestingly such a diet over a few weeks will change the bacteria living in our bowels which themselves send chemical massages to our brains to eat more healthy food. Previously, of course, other bacteria will have been sending messages asking for the unhealthy foods that they prefer. Amazingly our appetites are actually controlled by minute organisms in our bowels!

## Mediterranean diet

The Prevention with Mediterranean diet (PREDIMED) study of Dr Ramon Estruch of 7447 patients in Spain at high risk of heart disease found that those on a Mediterranean diet over the next five years had approximately 30 per cent fewer cardiac incidents (including death) than those on the traditional cardiologist's low fat diet. The results were so striking that independent ethical monitors stopped the trial for fear of damaging more patients on the cardiologist's diet after five years.

In the Mediterranean diet group, those patients who had an additional handful of hazel and walnuts each day experienced additional health benefit both physically and mentally.

## Depression and a Mediterranean diet

During the PREDIMED trial, 224 new cases of clinical depression were diagnosed by their general practitioners. There was a trend for a reduction in depression diagnoses in patients on the Mediterranean diet with extra nuts which became significant (almost half the numbers) in those with type 2 diabetes compared to the patients following the low fat diet.

What is not clear is whether the low-fat diet is harmful or the Mediterranean diet is positively healthy.

## BDNF

Possible health factors improved by a Mediterranean diet include increasing Brain Derived Neurotrophic Factor levels which are beneficial for brain health. The diet also reduces levels of inflammation which can be associated with harm to the brain. Increased BDNF levels stimulate new brain cell growth. Both exercise and preferably eating all our daily food in an eight-hour period enhance BDNF levels as does a period of reduced calorie intake once a week.

## Vitamin D

People who take supplements and vitamins in the long term die several years BEFORE others with one exception, vitamin D3.

In the UK and other northern countries the stores of vitamin D we make from the summer sun on our skin runs out at Christmas.

Depressed people tend to have lower vitamin D levels as they withdraw inside more out of the daylight. Low vitamin D levels can cause tiredness and even pains which will worsen symptoms of depression. In Britain the advice is to take vitamin D supplements from the end of September until April. People with dark skin should consider vitamin D supplements all year round.

## Healthy bowel flora

For many decades we have known that the microorganisms in the large bowel produce energy from digesting vegetable matter into acetic, propionic acid and butyric acid (the favourite food of the lining of our bowels themselves). A gorilla derives more than half of its daily energy requirements this way but dieticians tend to make no estimate of the calories involved in humans as they are not taught about the subject.

In the last ten years it has been discovered that almost 80 per cent of the micro organisms in human large bowels are new to human science and only recognisable from their DNA genetic imprint. Increasingly we realise that these organisms not only affect our nutrition but also our behaviour and mental state. The organisms are specialists for different foods and seem to be able to send messages to our brains saying 'Send more chocolate' 'Send more pasta'. This means that changing to a different healthy Mediterranean diet will meet with opposition from an unlikely source – your bowel microbiome. It often takes as long as six weeks before new organisms take over sending better messages to our brains 'Send more nuts and fish'!

# 12

# Dealing with avoidance, anger and other issues

## Dealing with avoidance

*Case study – Emma's story*

Emma had been married for two years when she discovered that she was pregnant for the first time. Like all mums-to-be, Emma and her husband were thrilled at the prospect of the arrival of a new baby. They decorated their spare bedroom as a nursery, and bought baby clothes, a pushchair and other baby equipment. They told all their friends about their expected new arrival. Emma, who was working as an auditor in a large financial company, decided that she was going to take a generous amount of maternity leave and asked her mother and mother-in-law to assist with childcare when she went back to work, at the same time making enquiries about having a part-time nanny.

Emma had an uneventful pregnancy, apart from some early morning sickness that abated after 12 weeks or so, and feeling tired in the second part of her pregnancy. However, from 30 weeks until she finished work when she was 37 weeks' pregnant, Emma felt well and full of energy. Just after she finished work, at 38 weeks, Emma's waters broke and, following the advice of her community midwife, she waited until her contractions were fairly frequent before going to hospital.

When she arrived at the hospital she was examined by a midwife and then a doctor and it quickly became clear that there was a major problem, as both midwife and doctor were unable to detect the baby's heartbeat. Emma and her husband reacted to this news with great shock, as all the antenatal checks had been perfectly normal and Emma had felt her unborn baby move just a few hours before her waters broke. Sadly, Emma delivered a stillborn daughter some hours later. To this day, despite a post mortem, no one has discovered the cause of the baby's death.

Very understandably, Emma was in a state of great shock and described feeling numb following this tragedy. She was discharged from hospital, but could not face going home to the house where the nursery had been prepared. Instead she went to stay with her mother. Other family members were helpful insofar as they were able to remove all the items prepared for the baby's arrival. However, Emma still felt unable to return to her house for several weeks.

Initially, she did not want to see anyone apart from her husband and her parents, and she stayed in bed for lengthy periods. She had many of the symptoms of PTSD, including having vivid and distressing dreams of the events at the hospital. She expressed feelings of guilt that she should have recognized that something was wrong with her pregnancy. These feelings of guilt persisted, despite reassurance from doctors that stillbirths sometimes occur for no reason that can be determined, and that there is nothing that one can do to prevent such tragedies. Many friends and relations tried to contact Emma to offer their condolences, but she avoided all contact with them.

After six weeks Emma decided she should go out with her husband to do the food shopping. However, on entering the supermarket the first thing she encountered was a young mother with her baby. Emma ran back to her car and went home. Although Emma was eventually able to see one or two close friends, she avoided any discussion of what had happened, and although her husband tried to encourage her to talk about her feelings of loss, she was unable to do this. Indeed, Emma displayed considerable irritability and feelings of anger and, on occasion, vented angry feelings towards her husband, without any particular trigger on his part.

Emma's employers contacted her, having been told of events by her husband. Their approach was very sympathetic; they simply said she was to take as much time as she needed to recover and that she should return to work if she wished in graduated steps. However, Emma knew that two women in her office were shortly due to give birth. For this reason, she decided that she could not return to work to face a situation with 'news of births and healthy babies'. She then announced that she was going to give in her notice. Her husband persuaded her not to do this.

It was at this point that Emma was referred to a therapist. At the assessment, Emma's overall presentation was one of considerable sadness, and over the four, long consultations that followed, she was able to begin to explain what had happened to her and talk about a very wide range of emotional responses. Later on she said that this was the first time she had 'really opened up'. By this time she recognized that she was doing anything to avoid talking about the tragedy. Being able to talk to her therapist then led to Emma talking to her husband. She explained some months after that 'opening up to someone she loved', although at first very difficult, led to feelings of enormous relief.

Emma, by this time, agreed with her therapist that tackling the avoidance behaviour was a priority. Nevertheless, it became clear that this avoidance needed to be tackled in small, graduated doses of difficulty. She and her therapist discussed a plan for breaking down her avoidance behaviours in a systematic way. Emma wrote down all the avoidances she had engaged in and arranged these in a hierarchy, so that the 'easier to manage' avoidance behaviours were at the bottom and the 'most difficult to manage' ones were at the top of the list. The most difficult task was visiting a work colleague who had just given birth to twins and being able to cradle one of the babies in her arms. At the bottom of the list of avoidance behaviours was the task of looking at pictures of babies on the Internet. In the middle of the list was the task of going to the supermarket on her own, having undertaken a preparatory visit in the company of her husband and looking out for mothers and babies.

Emma realized that all these tasks, aimed at exposing her to previously avoided situations, would cause her some distress. However, she realized that this was necessary in order to begin rebuilding her life. Indeed, although she found many of the exposure tasks difficult, once she had accomplished them she reported feeling much better.

A very important aspect of Emma's exposure was the development of a return to work plan. With her permission, her very understanding GP spoke, in strict confidence, to the company's occupational health adviser. Emma, with the support of her therapist, negotiated a return to work plan over a period of three months, so that she began working a few hours a day for three days a week and then building this time up, eventually returning to work on a full-time basis. Returning to work involved further exposure to some of the situations she had avoided, particularly speaking to colleagues who had just returned to work themselves after the birth of children.

By the time that she returned to work Emma still had some anxiety and periods of sadness. Emma and her husband decided, in our opinion very wisely, to put on hold trying for another child. Emma realized that a new baby would not, in any way, replace the daughter whose life had been lost just before birth. She also concluded that she needed more time to become stronger and work on developing ways of combating her anxiety and continuing distress. She and her husband still grieve for their daughter, who was buried in a local cemetery and whose grave they visit every week to lay flowers. As in the case of someone like Emma, one needs to have a plan for dealing with avoidance behaviours.

In summary it is important to recognize that avoidance of situations, thoughts or feelings only serves to perpetuate distress, and such avoidance can lead to more avoidance behaviour, so that life can become extremely restricted. If the exposure to previously avoided situations becomes unmanageable, you have tried too hard and perhaps too soon. If this is the case, stop and plan your exposure again. If the distress continues or gives rise to feelings or emotions that you consider to be overwhelming, please speak to your GP or – if you are receiving professional treatment – your doctor or therapist.

## Dealing with anger

Earlier on in this book (see Chapter 4), we told Joe's story and provided an account of Joe developing insight into the nature and reasons for his anger. He also became very aware of the potential results of anger in a road rage incident.

There are now a number of professional treatments available from the NHS (based on a cognitive behavioural approach), as well as anger management courses provided by the independent sector. In addition to becoming aware of the origins of anger, there are a number of components of anger management training offered by professionals. However, some of these components are suitable for individuals to apply as a self-help method.

One of the easiest strategies to deal with anger is to interrupt the anger by removing yourself, mentally or physically, from the situation. This requires you to become aware of when anger is likely to develop and how it might be triggered. The first step is to make a written list of these situations. Physically leaving the situation is obviously very effective if this can be achieved.

In the last few years it has become all too easy to respond to an email or Facebook message with an instant, angry response. You should therefore also make a pact with yourself to never respond immediately to any communication that upsets you.

It is also helpful to identify methods that might remove you from the situation by a process of mental distraction. As we saw in Joe's case, he was able to deal with his feelings of increased physical arousal by the use of meditation. Meditation is just one of a number of relaxation skills. The main difficulty for most people is the application of relaxation skills to real-life settings. For this reason it is usually very helpful to keep a diary record of successes and failures, so that you can learn from experience.

In therapies delivered by professionals, there is an emphasis on identifying the way in which people think about situations that evoke anger and also on identifying underlying assumptions. It may be, therefore, that you have some unhelpful attitudes. For example, you might come to recognize that your inclination is to believe that people should act in a way that suits you, rather than seeing that other people make choices of their own and that their choice may not be yours! You might also identify the unhelpful way in which your thoughts can be amplified. For example, you might react to an event that is a bit disappointing or frustrating by seeing it as catastrophic, rather than by letting the frustration or disappointment pass. Anger management also includes an emphasis on trying to see a range of situations in a different way; for example, for example very simply 'seeing the funny side of things' may serve to diffuse the anger.

If you receive CBT from a therapist to take more control of angry responses, there may be an emphasis on an acceptance that there are some things we cannot change. For example, children will always push the limits and at times say 'NO'. Alternatively, there are always going to be people who are going to think both politically and in many other ways quite differently from yourself. In addition, we need to follow the old maxim and 'forgive and forget', although this is much easier said than done. However, working on this, either as a self-help topic or in a professional therapy often yields good results.

Professional therapy may also include an approach called social skills training. Through treatment sessions, which use role play, one can learn to communicate more effectively and become more assertive, without displaying angry behaviours. This form of therapy focuses on learning new ways of verbal and non-verbal communication.

Anger and frustration are inevitable parts of human life. However, there is a range of methods for altering our responses, as demonstrated in Joe's story.

## Dealing with relationship problems

As we described in the case of Linda and Roy (see Chapter 5), whose marriage came to an end, the fundamental cause of the relationship breakdown was the couple's inability to communicate with each other. This was, of course, no fault of their own, but rather a reflection of the pain and anguish that they both felt but kept to themselves. It is therefore important to emphasize what we have mentioned above in several places in this book, that is, the need to talk and, particularly in the case of women and their partners, to talk to each other.

Providing detailed advice about relationship problems is outside of the scope of this book. However, there are many organizations who provide relationship support and facilitate the process of rebuilding a relationship after the tragedy of losing a baby. The best known charity in this area is Relate (<www.relate.org.uk>).

Relate has an excellent website, which provides information about the help that is available. We strongly recommend that those whose difficulties are similar to Linda and Roy's contact this, or a similar, organization to see what help may be available. If only one of you is prepared to do this, Relate and other organizations are still able to help and will willingly provide the appropriate counselling and advice.

## Dealing with sexual problems

As we described in the first part of this book, the loss of a baby often causes a breakdown in the sexual relationship between parents. Sometimes this is due to the relationship itself breaking down. If this is the case, there is obviously a need to try to resolve the relationship problems before attempting to deal with sexual problems. That said, sexual relationships are, of course, an important part of the way that we communicate with each other. We have described how sexual difficulties may arise because of low mood. If this is the situation, it is important to follow advice about improving mood (more of that in Chapter 14, in the section on behavioural activation).

There are some simple measures that one can take to deal with a wide variety of sexual problems. One of the difficulties often mentioned is a fear of failure if one attempts sexual activity. If this is the case, the couple often begin to avoid all physical contact, thus shutting down an important form of non-verbal communication. A suggested remedy for this is to make an initial ban on any sexual activity but, at the same time, to set time aside, on a daily basis, for non-sexual physical contact. It may be that holding hands or putting an arm around the shoulder is a good beginning. This might then progress to perhaps sitting to watch a film or television programme on the settee and maintaining physical contact. Another suggested route is to give each other a few minutes of massage, using massage oil or moisturizer, while at the same time remembering that sexual activity is banned. If this is clearly accepted by both partners, there is no fear of failure. Following a phase of non-sexual contact, one might progress to sexual contact without intercourse and gradually build one's confidence.

For many years now, sex therapy programmes provided by professionals have used this approach, with reports of considerable success. Simply put, taking away the source of the fear of failure is the effective ingredient. When one thinks about it, affectionate physical contact is something that virtually all of us need on a regular basis. Without this, we are inevitably going to feel isolated and, if our mood is already low, our mood will worsen.

Some couples may benefit from professional interventions; such interventions are available on the NHS and your GP can refer you. However, sex therapy is not available on the NHS in all areas and the amount of therapy that can be received is often limited. In many cases there is a need to find a sex therapist on a private basis, which will need to be paid for. A number of charities offer sex therapy at a reasonable rate and charge according to your ability to pay. Relate provides sex therapy for a fee. If you are seeking a sex therapist outside of the known, reputable charities, you need to ensure that the therapist is qualified and has received the appropriate training. They therefore need to be a member of the College of Sexual and Relationship Therapists (COSRT) or of the Institute of Psychosexual Medicine.

# 13

## Panic attacks

In Chapter 3 we told the first part of Ruth's story, which described her suffering her first panic attack four months after her baby Jonathan had died in her arms, aged seven days. Part 2 of Ruth's story follows and describes a short course of therapy, which led to Ruth recovering from her panic attacks.

### Case study – Ruth's story, part 2

Ruth was referred, by her GP, to the local Improving Access to Psychological Therapy (IAPT) service (for more information go to <https://www.england.nhs.uk/mental-health/adults/iapt/>). After a telephone assessment and a discussion about the form that the therapy would take, it was agreed that the following would help Ruth. First, it had become clear, in the course of the discussion with her GP, that Ruth would require some further help and support with respect to the loss of Jonathan. The therapist provided a list of support groups that Ruth might explore. Second, it was agreed that Ruth should also be provided with a short course of treatment for her panic attacks.

By the time the assessment took place, Ruth had suffered two more panic attacks, although these were not as severe as on the first occasion. In the meantime Ruth had also signed up to join a local Sands support group. The therapy for her panic attacks started with a detailed assessment process in which Ruth was able to tell her particular story and to say more about her background. She also completed some questionnaires, which she would repeat at the end of her therapy to see whether her treatment had been effective.

In the second session, the therapist explained the basis of the physical symptoms that Ruth was experiencing, and Ruth learned about the vicious cycle of anxiety (Figure 13.1). She came to understand that the trigger for her panic attack was the apprehension she felt about returning to work and meeting the woman who had had a healthy baby, born at about the same time as Jonathan. The therapist provided Ruth with some explanation about how apprehension produces physical symptoms (the 'fight or flight 'response) and how, in turn, the physical symptoms, are interpreted as a sign of a catastrophic physical illness (in Ruth's case, she thought she was having a heart attack). The therapist went on to explain that, as part of the 'fight or flight' response, her heart might beat very fast (up to twice or more rapidly than the normal resting heart rate).

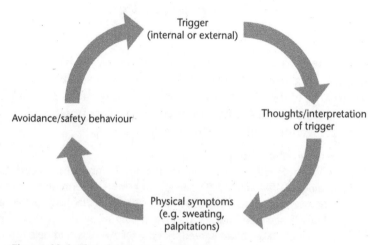

**Figure 13.1 The vicious cycle of anxiety**

Ruth also came to understand that, in addition to an increase in heart rate (which although frightening would cause no harm), her breathing began to increase in its rate, and that this was the body's way of preparing the individual for actual fight or flight. However, as no 'fight or flight' actually occurred, Ruth was in fact breathing in excess of requirements. This state of breathing in excess of bodily needs is called hyperventilation. Hyperventilation changes the body's chemical balance, causing a number of symptoms such as pins and needles, light-headedness, chest pain or discomfort and other panic symptoms. The experience of these symptoms then leads to a vicious cycle in itself, with physical symptoms causing catastrophic thoughts, and those catastrophic thoughts in turn producing more physical symptoms by increasing the 'fight or flight' response.

Ruth came to see that her escape from the supermarket had been her way of seeking safety and that, once she had been in the hands of the paramedic and the emergency department at the hospital, she felt reassured.

Ruth found this therapy session very helpful, as it explained what had happened to her that day in the supermarket during her lunch break. The therapist gave Ruth some written information, which described what had been discussed in the session and also suggested that she might find some resources on the No Panic website (<www.nopanic.org.uk>). The therapist explained that No Panic is the largest self-help charity for people who suffer panic attacks and anxiety. No Panic provides a very wide range of information, support and contact via social media and helplines.

The therapist devoted one session to discussing with Ruth possible triggers for her panic. During that session Ruth came to realize that there were a number of triggers in her case that might lead to a panic attack. She had particularly noticed that adverts on the television focusing on babies made her feel very uneasy. She was also anxious at the thought of visiting her cousin in Scotland in the months ahead. This was something that she feared because her cousin was in the early stages of pregnancy. After this session Ruth's homework was to make a list of all of the situations that she thought might trigger her to panic.

One session was devoted to dealing with Ruth's catastrophic thinking. Ruth had learned a lot through keeping the diary recommended by the therapist about the chain of thoughts accompanying panic. Following a discussion with her therapist Ruth identified some alternative ways of thinking. The therapist suggested that Ruth should use cue cards to remind herself of what she called 'thought challenges'. The cue cards, which Ruth kept in her handbag, simply contained irrational trigger thoughts followed by thoughts that she could use to challenge them. Ruth had a number of these cards; one said:

> If you are feeling light-headed and think that you are going to pass out, challenge this thought by remembering what you learned about overbreathing (hyperventilation). If you experience palpitations, you might think you are going to have a heart attack, but challenge this thought by thinking about the vicious cycle of anxiety.

In a subsequent session, the therapist helped Ruth to understand other principles of panic management. One of the sessions involved the therapist asking Ruth to breathe very quickly, so that she would be 'hyperventilating.' The therapist reassured Ruth that this was a very safe exercise and would show her how hyperventilation was producing the physical symptoms that can be so alarming in a panic attack. As her breathing rate increased Ruth very quickly began to feel light-headed and experienced an increase in her heart rate. Her therapist then instructed Ruth in a slow breathing exercise that quickly dispelled her physical symptoms. As 'homework', Ruth's therapist suggested that she try one of the very helpful breathing exercise apps available on the internet (for example, from <www.calm.com> – this particular app also provides some help with meditation, sleep and more general relaxation).

By the end of six therapy sessions, Ruth had a very good understanding of what panic attacks were. She had also learned some simple methods to control episodes of panic. After a discussion with her therapist, Ruth decided that she should take more steps to reduce her general state of tension and arousal by engaging in more physical exercise. She also decided that she should book herself on to a local meditation course.

Ruth's story illustrates the process of discovering what panic attacks are, how they develop and what triggers them – and then how panic can be controlled by efforts at breathing and relaxation, as well as by learning to deal with the catastrophic thoughts.

# 14

# Coping with depression and PTSD

Depressive symptoms are almost universal in people who have experienced tragic loss. More often than not, people with depressive symptoms – particularly those who have gone through a stillbirth or neonatal death – receive no help and do not use self-help methods.

We know that there are some very effective professional treatments for depression. Although there is still wide debate about the use and extent of antidepressant medication, there is no doubt that, for more severe states of depression, antidepressant drugs are a necessity for many people; they may also literally be life-saving because of the risk of suicide associated with severe depression. That said, many states of depression (particularly the mild to moderate forms) respond to self-help or to a combination of self-help with some limited professional contact.

The National Institute for Health and Care Excellence (NICE) in its latest review of evidence (NICE 2022) is currently updating its original guidance on the topic, published in 2009. For mild levels of depression, NICE guidance advises some common sense self-help approaches, including trying to improve sleep (see Chapter 11), and other 'low-intensity' interventions. The guidance also emphasizes the importance of physical activity and exercise (see Chapter 11).

The past two decades have seen a great increase in the use of self-help apps and CBT delivered via a computer. Although these programmes have become very popular, there remains a controversy about their effectiveness. Perhaps the best advice we can give you is as follows. It appears that some people do obtain a real benefit from the use of the computerized programmes and apps, although for others no benefit is obtained. Recent research has shown that some of these programmes work better if they are associated with some limited professional contact. It is also probably fair to say that, for severe levels of depression, these programmes are probably not helpful but, if the depression is mild to moderate, they may have some benefit. The NHS uses these methods widely.

One of the longest running and most popular computer delivered self-help methods comes from an Australian website: <https://moodgym.com.au>. This program was developed at the Australian National University in Canberra more than two decades ago, and was originally targeted at the very large number of people in Australia who did not have access to health professionals. However, research on its effectiveness demonstrated that anyone with lower levels of depression, with or without accompanying anxiety, might benefit. Registration on this website and access to its interactive programme is strictly anonymous and confidential, and there is considerable reassurance that any data you input to the web program will be handled with the highest levels of security. More than one million people, worldwide, have now accessed this site and used its modules.

The website contains information and questionnaires about the level of your mood, asks questions about feelings and thoughts, and then provides feedback. The programme involves a number of exercises based on CBT, which helps change thoughts, attitudes and behaviours. Sometimes MoodGYM is used in conjunction with professional help – for example, from a GP or a nurse practitioner – but more often is used only by the affected person. For many years, the website was free of charge, partly because it was sustained by government funding. However, in order to ensure that the website and all its resources can be sustained, a relatively small charge is made for each year's access.

## Professional treatments

This section refers to several pieces of guidance from NICE (below).

### NICE

- NICE – the National Institute for Health and Clinical Excellence – is an executive non-departmental public body that is part of the Department of Health in the UK. In the popular press, NICE is often referred to as the 'drugs-rationing body'. Although NICE does have an important role in determining which drugs can be prescribed by the NHS, it in fact has a much wider remit and publishes guidelines in four areas, covering:

- the use of health technologies within the NHS (such as the use of new and existing medicines, treatments and procedures);
- clinical practice (guidance on the appropriate treatment and care of people with specific diseases and conditions);
- guidance for public sector workers on health promotion and ill health avoidance;
- guidance for social care services and users.

NICE guidelines are published after extensive reviews of evidence and with input from medical professionals, representatives of patient and carer groups, and technical experts. Guidance is only finalized after extensive and wide-ranging consultation.

Some individuals require treatment from the GP or other health professionals. Excellent help is, as noted earlier in this book, available from midwives and health visitors. In the case of those whose distress continues the GP is the obvious first port of call. At this point the GP may advise that contact with Sands or a similar organization is the best source of help. However, GPs may initiate treatment themselves (principally with antidepressant medication) or may advise referral to specialist mental health services. This can include services specializing in the care and treatment of women who have particular problems during or after pregnancy, that is, perinatal mental health services.

## Perinatal mental health services

Ideally, professional treatment is best provided by those with experience and expertise in dealing with women whose difficulties occur in pregnancy, around the time of childbirth or during the period after this. It seems clear that these periods of time are associated with a number of unique characteristics. These include considerable changes in the endocrine (hormone) system. In addition, the social and psychological factors unique to pregnancy are of considerable importance.

Professionals in perinatal services will have considerable experience of maternity services and will know exactly how the maternity system works, particularly the role of various professionals. They will also have knowledge of some of the common physical conditions associated with pregnancy, childbirth and afterwards. In summary, the experience and skill level of perinatal services is very different from that of mental health professionals (doctors, nurses, social workers, occupational therapists, psychologists, and so on) who deal with a very diverse range of mental health problems.

Although people in some areas of the country have some access to perinatal mental health services, many areas of the country do not have such easy access. NHS England published a report by the Independent Mental Health Task Force in 2016. The report recognized these problems and noted (BMJ, 2018):

> One in five mothers suffers from depression, anxiety or in some cases psychosis during pregnancy or in the first year after childbirth. Suicide is the second leading cause of maternal death after cardiovascular disease. Mental health problems not only affect the health of mothers but can also have longstanding effects on children's emotional, social and cognitive development. The costs of perinatal and mental ill health are estimated at £8.1bn for each annual birth cohort, or almost £10,000 per birth. However, fewer than 15% of localities provide effective, specialist community perinatal services for women with severe or complex conditions, and more than 40% provide no service at all.

The UK government has committed to providing additional funding for specialist perinatal mental health services in all areas of England, aimed at allowing an additional 30,000 women each year to receive evidence based treatments closer to home when they need it. As well as providing additional funding, NHS England has appointed consultant perinatal psychiatrists to provide expert clinical guidance to the programme. Sadly, this area of mental health care, along with mental health services in general, is one where there is currently a need for considerable improvement.

## Treatments for depression

As noted above, NICE (2022) has published guidance on the care and treatment of individuals with depression and, certainly for milder levels of depression, the self-help methods described above may be of considerable assistance. NICE recommends a range of treatments for moderate and severe depression, defining moderate depression as: 'When a person has more symptoms that can make their daily life much more difficult than usual.' Severe depression is defined as: 'When a person has many symptoms that can make their daily life extremely difficult.' The guidance also points to the fact that a person may experience different levels of depression at different times.

NICE recommends that, before embarking on treatments with antidepressants, a person should try self-help and/or a programme of physical activity. However, if you do not respond to these simpler methods, you may be offered an antidepressant or a psychological treatment, or possibly a combination of anti-depressant and psychological treatment.

## The role of antidepressants

In general, antidepressant medications are being prescribed for an increasing number of people. Although, as the name implies, antidepressants are used to treat depressive states, they are also used in a very wide range of other conditions, including anxiety states, obsessive–compulsive disorder and PTSD. They are also used in a wide range of other non-psychiatric conditions – some classes of antidepressant medications are used routinely in the treatment of migraine, irritable bowel syndrome, chronic pain and premenstrual syndrome.

In 2022, some 86 million prescriptions were issued for anti-depressant medication, a rise of 21 million since 2016. By contrast there were 31 million prescriptions for antidepressants in 2006. There are various estimates of the number of people prescribed anti-depressants. When one considers the total number of prescrip-tions, one needs to take into account that some people will only receive one prescription, some will receive a number of prescrip-tions over the years, and others will receive a prescription over the entire year. However, there is a consensus that around 1 in 9 of the population will take an antidepressant in any one year, with widely varying rates across the UK. Perhaps understandably, rates of antidepressant medication prescription are higher in areas subject to socioeconomic deprivation.

Antidepressants were discovered shortly after the Second World War. The first antidepressant drugs belonged to a group called the monoamine oxidase inhibitors (usually referred to as MAOIs). This group of drugs works (as do all other antidepressants) on the neurotransmitters in the brain. However, it needs to be said that, even today after 60 years of research on the mechanism of action of antidepressants, we have no definitive knowledge of how they work. Since the MAOIs other drugs have been developed: first tricyclic antidepressants, and then about 25 years ago a group of drugs known as selective serotonin reuptake inhibitors (SSRIs), of which fluoxetine (Prozac) is probably the best known example. In addition to tricyclic antidepressants and SSRIs, a number of other closely related subtypes of antidepressant have also been developed.

It remains a mystery why two individuals presenting with the same symptoms of depression may react differently to the same antidepressant, one person apparently recovering in a textbook way from their depressive illness and the other appearing to not respond at all. Recent research has shown that individual genetic make-ups are responsible for these differences. Indeed, through a process of genetic testing, efforts are now being made to identify which antidepressant drugs will suit any particular individual. These developments are, of course, mirrored in general medicine, where there have been a number of advances in treating different types of illness – notably cancer – by matching the drug to the individual's specific genetic subtype. Reviews of the evidence have yielded complex results. Although, overall, as a very recent 'review of reviews' has shown that antidepressants are an important and effective treatment for significant levels of depression, some people appear to respond just as well to psychological treatments

What then of the role of antidepressants for those who have had a stillbirth or perinatal death? In our opinion, antidepressant medications can be very helpful. It is rather difficult to provide generalizations, as there is a need to consider all of the unique circumstances presenting. One example of where antidepressant medications may be necessary is that of someone who has a pre-existing history of recurring depressive episodes and has then suffered a further recurrence, triggered by the specific events surrounding the stillbirth or perinatal death. In another example, antidepressant medications can be considered when depressive symptoms do not resolve with the passage of time, particularly when suicidal thoughts are present. General practitioners are in a very difficult position as there are obvious limits to the time they are able to spend assessing an individual and, in some cases, the most appropriate course of action is to refer the person to the local perinatal psychiatry service.

## Psychological approaches

### CBT

In the introduction to Part 3, we described CBT as probably the most widely available therapy, and pointed to the NHS website. For depression, CBT involves focusing on thoughts, beliefs and attitudes and exploring the way these relate to how we behave. Depression is characterized by negative thoughts, which in turn can lead to negative behaviours, such as stopping things that give us pleasure. Treatment aims to identify and change negative patterns of thinking. The NHS delivers CBT for depression in two formats: a number of sessions in groups of 8–10 people, or individual CBT over a number of sessions.

### Interpersonal therapy

Interpersonal therapy has been shown to help some people with depression when this stems from relationships with family, partners and friends. Just like CBT, interpersonal therapy identifies how negative thoughts and attitudes arise from these relationships. The therapy follows a highly structured approach, often involving 12–16 sessions. Some evidence regarding Interpersonal therapy suggests that it works well in combination with antidepressant medication.

### Behavioural activation

One of the most important treatment approaches, and one that appears to be as effective as traditional CBT, is behavioural activation. This is particularly important as a means of self-help because the treatment method is – compared with many psychological therapies – very straightforward and easy to understand. We recommend an excellent book on behavioural activation at the end of this section. The approach is also recommended by NICE in their guidelines for the treatment of depression.

Behavioural activation focuses on poor levels of motivation, avoidance behaviour and loss of interest. More than 30 years ago an American psychologist, Charles Ferster, described a model of depression based on the principles of learning. Ferster simply observed that when people become depressed they use escape and avoidance of thoughts, feelings and various situations as a method of coping. Although in one sense this reduction in behaviour prevents people facing what they perceive as distressing, what also happens is that they begin to engage less with activities that give them pleasure and satisfaction. In psychological terms they receive less 'reinforcement' for coping from life in general, that is, from rewarding activities and pleasurable interactions with others. Quite simply, Ferster and others developed treatment approaches along the lines of increasing the amount of pleasurable and everyday behaviour and reducing avoidance. These are the approaches now called behavioural activation.

In recent years a number of research studies have shown that behavioural activation can be as effective as not only CBT, but also antidepressant medication. Behavioural activation has been used as a treatment method for people with all levels of depression – from mild to the most severe. Indeed, it is used in inpatient settings, where people with the most severe levels of depression receive treatment.

If you are going to use behavioural activation as a self-help approach, one of the most important issues is first to define your level of activity. This can be done by keeping a diary of what you do from day to day. Alongside this exercise you should also keep a record of what you have avoided each day and why you have avoided it. For example, you might have avoided going out to see a friend because you felt you could not cope, or that you might let yourself down in some way and your friend would think badly of you. More specifically, you might record that you don't go out to meet a friend because you 'can't be bothered'. Thus keeping a diary of what you do and what you avoid is a really good starting point.

Once you have kept a diary for a few days, you might then list all the things that you used to do that you now no longer do or do much less often. This might include avoiding the cinema, turning down invitations to parties and functions, not going shopping, not going to a yoga class, not going line dancing, not going to a book club, not walking for pleasure or not inviting friends home. This way you have a good picture of the current situation and a good picture of what 'normal' life and activities might look like. Central to this method is the therapist discussing this with you to, in a sense, help you to help yourself. If you are using behavioural activation as a self-help method, you should share this section of the book with a family member or friend – someone who might work with you to put behavioural activation into action.

The next stage in behavioural activation is a process called activity scheduling. At its simplest, activity scheduling means increasing your level of behaviour, in a graduated way over a number of weeks and trying, one by one, to engage in behaviours you have either avoided or are doing much less often. One of the most important principles here is to list these avoided behaviours in a hierarchical form, that is, with those that are most difficult to achieve at the top, and those easier to achieve at the bottom of the list. You should then try to tackle behaviours from the bottom of the list and, in increasing doses of difficulty over days and weeks, work your way up the hierarchy.

It is very important to pace yourself realistically. Do not try to do too much too soon, but use the principle of not only doing things in a graduated way, but also tackling tasks that are difficult but manageable. Trying to do too much too soon may lead to a worsening sense of failure and thoughts such as, 'I knew I could never overcome this problem.' If you have a family member or friend to help, he or she may be able to help you judge the speed at which you increase your level of activity and support and encourage you through setbacks. Indeed, it is extremely unusual to complete a course of behavioural activation without experiencing one or more setbacks.

Continuing to keep a diary is very important in monitoring progress. It is always helpful to look back over the past days and weeks to reflect on how much progress has been made. It is also important to see how your thinking has changed and whether your predictions have been realized – for example, that going out with a friend will lead to a number of negative consequences. What usually happens is that you find that exposing yourself to situations you have avoided will help show you that your expectations were wrong, and thus disprove your worst fears.

If you are to embark on a programme of behavioural activation without the help of a therapist, we recommend that you use *Manage Your Mood* by Professor David Veale and Dr Rob Willson, which will serve as a very helpful resource (Veale and Willson, 2007).

## PTSD

NICE recommends two treatments with the best evidence to support their use in PTSD, and these psychological treatments are specific for individuals with this condition. These are:

- Trauma-focused CBT
- Eye movement desensitization and reprocessing (EMDR).

NICE (2018) describes these treatments as follows.

### Trauma-focused CBT:

A psychological treatment for PTSD based on cognitive behavioural therapy (CBT). CBT focuses on a person's distressing feelings, thoughts (or 'cognitions') and behaviour and helps to bring about a positive change. In trauma-focused CBT, the treatment concentrates specifically on the memories, thoughts and feelings that a person has about the traumatic event.

If you are offered this treatment, your healthcare professional will encourage and help you to gradually recall and think about the trauma. This can be done in various ways including listening to recordings of your own account of the trauma.

You will be given help to cope with any emotional distress and behavioural problems that may arise during treatment.

As the painful and traumatic memories begin to decrease, you may be encouraged and helped to start activities that you have been avoiding since the trauma, such as driving a car if you have avoided driving since an accident.

### EMDR

This is another psychological treatment for PTSD in which a healthcare professional will help you to identify key memories of the trauma (including all of the negative thoughts, feelings and sensations experienced at the time of the event). EMDR aims to change how you feel about these memories and helps you to have more positive emotions, behaviour and thoughts.

During EMDR, you will be asked to concentrate on an image connected to the traumatic event and the related negative emotions, sensations and thoughts, while paying attention to something else, usually the therapist's fingers moving from side to side in front of your eyes. After each set of eye movements (about 20 seconds), you should be encouraged to let go of the memories and discuss the images and emotions that you experienced during the eye movements. This process is repeated, this time with a focus on any difficult, persisting memories. Once you feel less distressed about the image, you should be asked to concentrate on it while having a positive thought relating to it. It is hoped that through EMDR you can have more positive emotions, thoughts and behaviour in the future.

You may find it helpful to read Kevin Gournay's book on PTSD, *Coping with Post Traumatic Stress Disorder* (Gournay, 2015).

## Coping with the consequences of use of alcohol and other drugs

Perhaps the most important step in dealing with the excessive use of alcohol or the use of other drugs is to be honest. In the first instance this may be a question of being honest with one's self, as admitting to others that there may be a problem is often very difficult. With regard to alcohol there are certainly many things that one can do about an increase in alcohol intake, beginning with attempts to adhere to the advice given by the UK Chief Medical

Officers. The latest guidance can be found at: <https://assets. publishing.service.gov.uk/media/5a7f51b4e5274a2e87db5206/ summary.pdf>. This provides detailed advice and the reasons for providing this advice.

## On regular drinking

New weekly guideline (*this applies for people who drink regularly or frequently, i.e. most weeks*)

The Chief Medical Officers' guideline for both men and women is that:

- To keep health risks from alcohol to a low level, it is safest not to drink more than 14 units a week on a regular basis. A unit is one small glass of wine (90 ml), one half-pint or a bottle of 4.0% beer, or one single(pub) measure of spirits.
- If you regularly drink as much as 14 units per week, it is best to spread your drinking evenly over three or more days. If you have one or two heavy drinking episodes a week, you increase your risks of death from long-term illness and from accidents and injuries.
- The risk of developing a range of health problems (including cancers of the mouth, throat and breast) increases the more you drink on a regular basis.

A good way to cut down the amount you drink is to have several drink-free days each week. In addition there are some other simple strategies that you can use to reduce your alcohol intake, for example drinking more slowly, and alternating alcoholic drinks with water or soft drinks. You also need to plan just how much and when you are going to drink on a social occasion. The success rate of these simple self-help measures is increased if someone with whom you have a trusting relationship knows what you are doing. Often both women and their partners are drinking excessively. Therefore, there is a need to have an agreement about matters such as the week's shopping and whether or not you buy that extra bottle of wine to drink with a meal.

Please remember that, in the long term, even small amounts of alcohol act as a depressant and may serve to magnify already existing problems. If self-help does not work and the problems escalate, it is important to seek professional help. The GP is, of course, the first port of call.

Some people benefit from attending one of the widely available self-help groups, such as Alcoholics Anonymous (AA – <www.alcoholics-anonymous.org.uk>) It is worth noting that AA meetings can benefit people with a wide range of alcohol problems and that one does not need to be drinking very large amounts to find these meetings helpful. Meetings are widely available, cost nothing and, as the name implies, strictly anonymous. AA also offers 'open meetings' to the general public – anyone may attend these irrespective of whether or not they are drinking too much.

The NHS now runs a range of community alcohol services. It is worth noting that these services are now somewhat different in England and Wales, as opposed to Scotland. The NHS website provides information and advice on this topic (see <https://www.nhs.uk/live-well/alcohol-support/>).

Over the past few years, the use of illicit drugs has become more common. Drugs such as cannabis are freely available. The cost of drugs is, by any standards, modest, getting 'high' costing much less than an evening in the pub. Although there is considerable controversy about cannabis, particularly the pros and cons of whether its use should be legal, in the author's experience cannabis use is very detrimental to those who are undergoing emotional turmoil following stillbirth or perinatal death. As with alcohol there is often short-term relief of distress but, following this short-term relief, there is often an increased level of emotional turmoil. The NHS offers a range of services for people who have problems with illicit drugs. A summary of what is available may be found at NHS: drug addiction: getting help.

## Other conditions

Above we have described what we consider to be the most common problems associated with stillbirth and perinatal death, but that is not to say that our account is exhaustive. There are now many psychological treatments with proven effectiveness for a range of disorders, including general anxiety and obsessive–compulsive disorder. Most of these treatments use psychological approaches, principally involving CBT. However, for some conditions, such as severe obsessive–compulsive disorder, treatment with medication is also employed alongside psychological treatments. For more information about obsessive compulsive disorder, see Gournay, Piper and Rogers (2012).

If you are affected by a mental health problem that has not been mentioned in this book, we recommend that you visit the NHS website. In addition, for more detail of treatments and their effectiveness, carry out an Internet search using the terms 'NICE' and the name of the mental health problem you require more information on.

# Conclusion

At the beginning of this book we stated our aim as being to provide information and advice to women and their partners who have been affected by the loss of a baby by stillbirth or death in the days soon after birth. Although the authors have many years of experience of providing care and treatment, our experience of writing has brought back many memories of individuals who have been deeply affected by this tragedy. Their lives, it is fair to say, will have changed forever because of their loss.

Writing this book has also caused us to reflect on the care provided at the time the loss occurred and the care and treatment provided afterwards. We are aware that many women and their partners go on to suffer without professional help or support for days, weeks, months or even years; their lives and the lives of their families may be affected in many different ways. We are also aware that for many women, and their partners, whose problems have been identified, care and treatment could be much improved.

We have described the difficulty of accessing perinatal mental health services. These services employ professionals with considerable specialist skills and expertise and, of central importance, the right set of attitudes to their job. In our view, as with those who care for people in their last days and weeks of life, you need to be a special person to do this job. It is our belief that these special people do exist, and that the barriers to providing decent perinatal mental health services to all those who require this expertise boils down to one matter – that of resources. We are both realists, because we have considerable experience of the NHS and know that there will never be enough resources to deal with all health problems in the population, particularly because of a changing demographic. However, it is our belief that the stillbirth and neonatal loss have insufficient weight given to them as a priority.

Brenda has identified the shortage of midwives and indicated that training in this area could be improved, and we have both identified the need for improvement of perinatal mental health services. Perhaps now what is needed is an effective campaign to ensure that the thousands of women and their partners and families (a population in much need) are able to access the care and treatment they require.

# Useful addresses and online resources

## Useful addresses

**Abbie's Fund**
Raises money to provide memory boxes to local hospitals. Offers financial support to bereaved parents.
Email: infor@abbiesfund.co.uk
Tel: 07788 568388

**Abigail's Footsteps**
Charity supporting midwives and families coping with stillbirth.
Email: infor@abigailsfootsteps.co.uk
Tel: 01634 225145

**Aching Arms**
Charity supporting those who have lost a baby at any stage of pregnancy, at birth or shortly afterwards.
Email: info@achingarms.co.uk
Tel: 07876504042

**Action on Pre-eclampsia**
Supporting women and families by increasing public awareness. Campaigns for research and offers specialist training for professionals to enable them to detect and manage the condition better.
Email: info@apec.org.uk
Tel: 020 8427 4217

**Aidan's Elephants**
Supports Airedale NHS Trust caring for bereaved parents and families. Donating Life Certificates and other memorials and advice and midwife bereavement training.
Email: aidanselephants@gmail.com

**Alcoholics Anonymous (AA)**
Website: www.alcoholics-anonymous.org.uk
Tel: 0800 7697555

**Antenatal Results and Choices (ARC)**
Offers information and support to parents before and after antenatal screening, when their baby has an anomaly and making difficult and painful decisions. Also provides bereavement support.
Email: info@arc-uk.org
Tel: 0207 713 7356

**Baby Lifeline**
Charity supporting pregnant women and newborn babies, raising funds to provide equipment and training maternity support workers.
Email: info@babylifeline.org.uk
Tel: 01676 534 671

**BLISS**
Supports parents of premature or sick babies and raises funds to help to care for the babies.
Email: hello@bliss.org.uk
Tel: 0808 801 0322

**Cariad Angel Gowns (for stillborn and neonatal loss)**
Takes donated wedding gowns and transforms them into burial outfits. Provides memory packs for those suffering loss through miscarriage, ectopic, stillbirth or neonatal loss. Provides a Life Certificate for those not eligible for a birth or death certificate.
Email: cariadan@cariadangelgowns.org.uk

**Ectopic Pregnancy Trust**
Raises awareness of ectopic pregnancy and early pregnancy complication and provides support and information.
Email: ept@ectopic.org,.uk
Tel: 0207733 2653

**4 Louis**
Charity providing memory boxes to bereaved parents and support.
Website: www.4louis.co.uk

**Group B Strep Support**
Provides evidence-based information to families and health professionals. Dedicated to eradicating group B strep infections, including meningitis in babies.
Email: info@gbss.org.uk
Tel: 01444 416176

**ICP Support**
Charity for intrahepatic cholestasis of pregnancy, raising awareness of the condition and support for women affected by the condition.
Email: admin@icpsupport.org
Tel: 0121 323 4316

**Jude Brady Foundation**
Raises awareness of stillbirth and neonatal death and provides funds for child-related good causes.
Email: Nicola@judebradyfoundation.co.uk
Tel: 01473 375034

**Kicks Count**
Provides education on the importance of monitoring the unborn baby movements for parents and professionals.
Email: info@kickscount.org.uk
Tel: 07403 656611

**Life after Loss**
Helps anyone affected by the loss of a baby at any stage of pregnancy or early life for any reason.
Email: Helen@lifeafterloss.org.uk
Tel: 02892 605578

**Lily Mae Foundation**
Supports parents and families affected by stillbirth or neonatal loss.
Email: info@lilymaefoundation.org
Tel: 07853 060073

**Little Things and Co.**
Provides emotional and practical support to anyone affected by the loss of a baby. Provides clothing for any gestation, practical items and a support group.
Email: info@ltandco.org

**Lullaby Trust**
Raises awareness of Sudden Infant Death Syndrome (SIDS) and provides advice on sleep for babies and support for bereaved families.
Website: www.lullabytrust.org.uk
Tel: 0808 802 6868

## Making Miracles
Provides support and counselling for families of high-risk pregnancies and those who have suffered loss. Provides specialist equipment to identify symptoms earlier.
Email: Kelly@makingmiracles.org.uk
Tel: 07791872115

## MAMA Academy
Charity that promotes stillbirth prevention strategies, giving parents up-to-date information about when to call the maternity team. Accredited by the Royal College of Midwives.
Email: contact@mamaacademy.org.uk
Tel: 07427 851670

## Miscarriage And Stillborn Support (MASS)
Supports and provides counselling for those who have suffered the loss of a baby through miscarriage or stillbirth.
Email: massmanagement.uk@gmail.com
Tel: 01234 219909

## The Midlands and North of England Stillbirth Study (MiNESS)
Study funded by Sands (Stillbirth and Neonatal Death Society) in partnership with Action Medical Research, Cure Kids and Tommy's. It is the largest of four similar studies into the cause of stillbirth, which all report the same findings.
Website: https://clinicaltrials.gov/ct/show/NCT02025530

## Miscarriage Association
Provides support and information for anyone affected by miscarriage, ectopic pregnancy or molar pregnancy.
Email: infor@miscarriageassociation.org.uk
Tel: 01924 200799

## Mariposa Trust
Supports anyone who has lost a baby at any stage of pregnancy, birth or infancy, whether the loss is recent or historic.
Email: support@sayinggoodbye.org
Tel: 0845 293 8027

## Miscarriage Information Support Service (MISS)
Support group for women and partners who have suffered a miscarriage.
Email: miscarriageinfosuppservice@gmail.com
Tel: 07702464874

**National Maternity Support Foundation (NMSF), also known as Jake's Charity**
Set up following a tragic stillbirth when the nearest maternity unit was closed. Campaigns to help keep maternity services available and accessible.
Email: info@jakescharity.org

**Parkrun**
Website: www.parkrun.org
Junior events are at: www.parkrun.org.uk/events/juniorevents/

**Petals**
Charity providing free counselling for women and partners suffering psychological distress from trauma and grief related to pregnancy loss.
Email: contact@petalscharity.org
Tel: 0300 688 0068

**Pregnancy Crisis Care (Plymouth & SE Cornwall)**
Provides counselling for any pregnancy-related crises, miscarriage, still-birth, neonatal death, ectopic pregnancy or therapeutic termination of pregnancy for medical reasons within Plymouth and the surrounding areas.
Email: contact@pregnancycrisiscare.org.uk

**Relate**
Charity providing relationship support throughout the UK. Services include counselling for couples, families, young people and individuals, sex therapy, mediation and training courses.
Website: www.relate.org.uk

**Stillbirth and Neonatal Death Society (Sands)**
Charity that supports anyone who has been affected by the death of a baby before, during or shortly after birth and also miscarriage. Also provides support groups.
Website: www.uk-sands.org/
Email: helpline@uk-sands.org
Tel: 0808 164 3332

**Sands Lothians**
In the Edinburgh and West Lothian areas provides emotional and practical support following miscarriage, stillbirth or loss soon after birth.
Email: info@sands-lothians.org.uk
Tel: 0131 622 6263

### Spinal Muscular Atrophy Support Group

Provides practical advice and support for parents of babies from diagnosis through the days ahead. Babies with type 1 of this condition rarely survive their first birthday.
Email: supportservices@smasupportuk.org.uk
Tel: 01789 267520

### Scottish Cot Death Trust

Provides bereavement support counselling following the sudden unexpected death of a baby or young child.
Email: contact@scottishcotdeatgtrust.org
Tel: 0141 357 3946

### SiMBA

Helps families gather precious items for the memory box and provides a support group.
Email: events@simbacharity.org.uk
Tel: 01368 860 141

### Our Missing Peace

Campaign to help all bereaved parents find support as quickly as possible.
Email: ourmissingpeace@outlook.com

### Teddy's Wish

Raises funds for potentially life-saving research into SIDS (sudden infant death syndrome), stillbirth and neonatal death and supports grieving families.
Email: Jennifer@teddyswish.org
Tel: 07813133787

### Time Norfolk

Charity providing support for anyone affected by pregnancy loss, miscarriage, stillbirth, ectopic pregnancy termination or infertility and pre- and postnatal depression.
Email: info@timenorfolk.org.uk
Tel: 01603 482732

### The Last Kiss Foundation

Founded to help bereaved families and give financial help to ensure no baby is buried in an unidentified grave.
Email: info@thelastkissfoundation.co.uk
Tel: 07814 660742

**Together for Short Lives**
Charity for children with life-threatening and life-limiting conditions and support for their families.
Email: myra.johnson@togetherforshortlives.org.uk
Tel: 0117 989 7820

**Tommy's Charity**
Supports research into early and late miscarriage and provides information and support for parents.
Website: www.tommys.org/
Tel: 0207 398 3400

**Twins and Multiple Births Association**
A charity supporting all multiple birth families, and a support group for parents who have lost a child.
Email: support-team@tamba.org.uk

## Online resources

**Calm**
Information on breathing, meditation, sleep and more general relaxation.
Website: www.calm.com

**FAST**
Self-administered test for problem drinking.
Website: www.verywellmind.com/the-fast-alcohol-screening-test-69495

**HelpGuide**
A guide to mental and emotional health.
Website: www.helpguide.org

**Mental Health Foundation**
Markets an online mindfulness course for a small sum.
Website: www.mentalhealth.org.uk/a-to-z/m/mindfulness

**Michigan Alcohol Screening Test**
This is available on the internet at no charge.
Website: lttp://counsellingresource.com/lib/quizzes/drug-testing/alcohol-mast

**MoodGYM**
One of the longest running and most popular computer delivered self-help methods for promoting good mental health comes from an Australian website.
Website: https://moodgym.com.au

**NHS**
Website: www.nhs.uk

**Dr Michael Beary**
mikebeary.blogspot.com

**No Panic**
Website: www.nopanic.org.uk

**Safe drinking guidance**
The UK Chief Medical Officer's latest guidance on safe drinking.
Website: www.gov.uk/government/publications/alcohol-consumption-advice-on-low-risk-drinking

# References and further reading

American Psychiatric Association (2013) *Diagnostic and Statistical Manual of Mental Disorders* (5th ed.). Washington, DC.

Ashcroft, B., Elstein, M., Boreham, N. and Holm, S. (2003) 'Midwives on the labour ward', *BMJ*, 327:571–630.

Beck, J.S. (2011) *Cognitive Behavior Therapy: Basics and Beyond*. New York: Guilford Press.

Births and Deaths Registration Act (1953) Available online at: <https://www.legislation.gov.uk/ukpga/Eliz2/1-2/20>.

BMJ (2018) 'Depression in adults: campaigners and doctors demand full revision of NICE guidance'. Available online at: <www.bmj.com/content/361/bmj.k2681>.

Chatterjee, R. (2017) *The 4 Pillar Plan*. London: Penguin.

Chief Coroner UK (2023) Guidance No. 45. 'Stillbirth and Live Birth Following Termination of Pregnancy'.

Gournay, K. (2015) *Coping with Post Traumatic Stress Disorder*. London: Sheldon Press.

Gournay, K, Piper, R. and Rogers, P. (2012) *Coping with Obsessive Compulsive Disorder*. London: Sheldon Press.

Healthline (2016) 'Alcohol, drugs and babies: do you need to worry?'. Available online at: <www.healthline.com/health/pregnancy/alcohol-drugs#overview1>.

Ismail, K. M. K. and Kilby, M. D. (2003) 'Human parvovirus B19 infection and pregnancy'. *Obstetrician & Gynaecologist*, 5:4–9. Available online at: <http://onlinelibrary.wiley.com/doi/10.1576/toag.5.1.4/pdf>.

Kirkup, B. (2013) 'The report of the Morecambe Bay Investigation: An independent investigation into the management, delivery and outcomes of care provided by the maternity and neonatal services at the University Hospitals of Morecambe Bay NHS Foundation Trust from January 2004 to June 2013'. Available online at: <www.gov.uk/government/publications>.

*The Lancet* (2016) 'Ending Preventable Stillbirths Series Study Group'. Volume 387. Available online at: <http://www.thelancet.com/pb/assets/raw/Lancet/stories/series/stillbirths2016-exec-summ.pdf>.

MAPPG (2015), Mindful Nation UK: Report by the Mindfulness All-Party Parliamentary Group. Available at: <https://themindfulnessinitiative.org.uk/images/reports/Mindfulness-APPG-Report_Mindful-Nation-UK_Oct2015.pdf>.

MBRRACE-UK (2016b) 'Mothers and babies: reducing risk through audits and confidentiality enquiries across the UK. (MBRRACE-UK)'. Available online at: <www.npeu.ox.ac.uk/mbrrace-uk/pmrt>.

MBRRACE-UK (2023a) *Perinatal Mortality Surveillance Report. UK Perinatal Deaths for Births from January to December 2014*. Oxford: MBRRACE-UK.

MBRRACE-UK (2023b) Maternal, Newborn and Infant Clinical Outcome Review Programme: A Comparison of the Care of Black and White Women Who Have Experienced a Stillbirth or Neonatal Death.

MBRRACE-UK (2023c) Maternal, Newborn and Infant Clinical Outcome Review Programme: A Comparison of the Care of Asian and White Women Who Have Experienced a Stillbirth or Neonatal Death.

MedicinePlus (2017) 'Pregnancy and herpes'. Available online at: <http://medlineplus.gov/ency/article/001368.htm>.

MiNESS (2017) 'The Midlands and North of England Stillbirth Study (MiNESS)'. Available online at: <https://clinicaltrials.gov/ct/show/NCT02025530>.

National Pregnancy in Diabetes Audit (2014) National Pregnancy in Diabetes Audit Report, 2014. England, Wales and the Isle of Man. Available online at: <www.hquip.org.uk>.

NHS (2015a) 'Overview. stillbirth'. Available online at: <www.nhs.uk/conditions/Stillbirth/Pages/Definition.aspx>.

NHS (2015b) 'What are the risks of group B streptococcus (GBS) infection during pregnancy?' Available online at: <www.nhs.uk/chq/pages/2037.aspx?categoryid=54>.

NHS (2015c) 'Listeriosis'. Available online at: <www.nhs.uk/conditions/Listeriosis/Pages/Introduction.aspx>.

NHS (2015d) 'Rubella (German measles)'. Available online at: <www.nhs.uk/chq/Pages/1104.aspx>.

NHS (2015e) 'Cytomegalovirus (CMV)'. Available online at: <www.nhs.uk/chq/Pages/1108.aspx?CategoryID=54>.

NHS (2016a) 'What are the risks of chickenpox during pregnancy?' Available online at: <www.nhs.uk/chq/Pages/1109.aspx?CategoryID=5>.

NHS (2016b) 'What are the risks of toxoplasmosis during pregnancy?' Available online at: <www.nhs.uk/chq/pages/1107.aspx?CategoryID=54>.

NHS (2017a) 'Mindfulness training may help you keep the weight off'. Available online at: <www.nhs.uk/news/food-and-diet/mindfulness-training-may-help-you-keep-weight>.

NHS (2017b) 'Why are pregnant women at higher risk of flu complications?' Available online at: <www.nhs.uk/chq/Pages/3096.aspx?CategoryID=5>.

NHS (2017c) 'Whooping cough vaccination in pregnancy'. Available online at: <www.nhs.uk/conditions/pregnancy-and-baby/pages/whooping-cough-vaccination-pregnant.aspx#advised>.

NICE (2008) 'Antenatal care. Routine care for the healthy pregnant woman'. Available online at: <https://www.rcog.org.uk/en/guidelines-research-services/guidelines/antenatal-care/>.

NICE (2018) 'Post-traumatic stress disorder: management'. NG116. Available online at: <http://www.nice.org.uk/guidance/ng116>.

NICE (2018) 'Depression in adults: recognition and management'. NG222. Available online at: <http://www.nice.org.uk/guidance/ng222>.

NICE (2019) 'Hypertension in pregnancy: diagnosis and management'. NG133. Available online at: <http://www.nice.org.uk/guidance/ng133>

NICE (2022) 'Parvovirus B19 infection'. Clinical knowledge summaries. Available online at: <https://cks.nice.org.uk/parvovirus-b19-infection#!scenariorecommendation:10>.

NPEU (2018) 'MBRRACE-UK perinatal mortality reporting tool'. Available online at: <www.npeu.ox.ac.uk/mbrrace-uk/pmrt>.

Office for National Statistics (2021) 'Provisional births in England and Wales'. Available online at: <http://www.ons/gove.uk>.

RCM (2008) 'Registration of stillbirths and certification for pregnancy loss before 24 weeks' gestation'. Available online at: <www.rcm.org.uk/news-and-views-and-analysis/analysis/registration>.

RCM (2016a) 'State of maternity services report 2016'. Available online at: <https://www.rcm.org.uk/sites/default/files/ENGLAND%20SOMS%202018%20-%20FINAL%20%2803.09.2018%29.pdf>.

RCM (2016b) 'News. Budget cuts, service cuts, staffing shortages = maternity services in 2016'. Available online at: <https://www.rcm.org.uk/news-views-and-analysis/news/budget-cuts-service-cuts-staffing-shortages-maternity-services-in-2016>.

RCM (2017a) 'The gathering storm: England's midwifery workforce challenges'. Available online at: <https://www.rcm.org.uk/sites/default/files/The%20gathering%20storm%20-%20Englands%20midwifery%20workforce%20challenges%20A5%2020pp_3.pdf>.

RCM (2017b) 'Survey results about the health, safety and wellbeing of midwives working in education. RCM Caring for You Campaign'. Available online at: <https://www.rcog.org.uk/en/guidelines-research-services/guidelines/gtg10a/>.

RCM (2017c) 'Half UK units closed their doors'. Available online at: <www.rcm.org.uk/news-views-and-analysis/news/'half-uk-units-closed-their-doors'>.

RCM (2021) 'RCM warns of midwife exodus as maternity staffing crisis grows'. Available online at: <https://www.rcm.org.uk/media-releases/2021/september/rcm-warns-of-midwife-exodus-as-maternity-staffing-crisis-grows/>.

RCM (2023) 'England state of maternity services'. Available online at: <https://www.rcm.org.uk/media/6915/england-soms-2023.pdf>.

RCOG (2006) 'The management of severe pre-eclampsia/eclampsia. Guideline No. 10 (A)'. Available online at: <https://www.rcog.org.uk/en/guidelines-research-services/guidelines/gtg10a/>.

RCOG (2010) 'Late intrauterine fetal death and stillbirth'. Green Top Guideline no. 55. Available online at: <https://www.rcog.org.uk/en/guidelines-research-services/guidelines/gtg55/>.

RCOG (2011a) 'Antepartum haemorrhage'. Green Top Guideline no. 63. Available online at: <https://www.rcog.org.uk/en/guidelines-research-services/guidelines/gtg63/>.

RCOG (2011b) 'Placenta praevia, Placenta praevia accreta and vasa praevia: diagnosis and management'. Green Top Guideline no. 27. Available online at: <https://www.rcog.org.uk/en/guidelines-research-services/guidelines/gtg27/>.

RCOG (2012a) 'Information for you. When your baby dies before birth'. Available online at: <https://www.rcog.org.uk/en/patients/patient-leaflets/when-your-baby-dies-before-birth/>.

RCOG (2012b) 'Information for you. Pre-eclampsia'. Available online at: <https://www.rcog.org.uk/globalassets/documents/patients/patient-information-leaflets/pregnancy/pi-pre-eclampsia.pdf>.

RCOG (2013) 'Group B streptococcus (GBS) infection in newborn babies'. Available online at: <www.northerntrust.hscni.net/pdf/Group_B_streptococcus_(GBS)_infection_in_newborn_babies.pdf>.

RCOG (2014) 'Umbilical cord prolapse'. Green Top Guideline no. 50. Available online at: <https://www.rcog.org.uk/en/guidelines-research-services/guidelines/gtg50/>.

RCOG (2015) 'Revised guideline on chickenpox in pregnancy published'. Available online at: <https://www.rcog.org.uk/en/news/rcog-release-revised-guideline-on-chickenpox-in-pregnancy-published/>.

Sands (2007) 'Forms and certificates'. Available online at: <www.sands.org.uk/forms-and-certificates>.

Sands (2016a) 'Pregnancy loss and the death of a baby. Guidelines for professionals. 4th Edition'. Available at: <www.sands.org.uk/professionals/bereavement-care-resources/sands-guidelines-4th-edition>.

Sands (2016b) 'Family support pack'. Available at: <www.sands.org.uk/support-you/how-we-offer-support/family-support-pack>.

Vance, M. E. (2009) 'The placenta'. In Fraser, D. M. and Cooper, M. A. (eds), *Myles Textbook for Midwives*, 15th edn. London: Churchill Livingstone. Page 152.

Veale, D. and Willson, R. (2007) *Manage Your Mood: How To Use Behavioral Activation Techniques To Overcome Depression*. London: Constable & Robinson.

Wikipedia (2017a) 'Medical education in the United Kingdom'. Available online at: <http://en.wikipedia.org/wiki/Medical_education_in_the_United_Kingdom>.

Wikipedia (2017b) 'Chorioamnionitis'. Available online at: <https://en.wikipedia.org/wiki/Chorioamnionitis>.

Wooller, S. (2023) 'Lack of staff forced four in ten NHS maternity units to turn away expectant mothers last year, alarming investigation reveals'. Mail Online, at: https://www.dailymail.co.uk/news/article-11823625/Lack-staff-forced-four-ten-NHS-maternity-units-turn-away-expectant-mothers-year.htmls>.

World Health Organisation (1992) *International Statistical Classification of Diseases and Related Health Problems*, 10th Revision (ICD-10). Geneva: WHO.

World Health Organization (2019) *International Statistical Classification of Diseases: The Global Standard for Diagnostic Health Information*, 11th Revision (ICD-11). Geneva: WHO.

# Index

## Join the Sheldon Press community today, sign up for our newsletter!

- Select a **FREE eBook** or extract to read upon joining

- Keep up with our latest publishing and exciting author news

- Be the first to hear about book prize draws, free extracts, and upcoming author events

Simply scan the QR code below or head to www.sheldonpress.co.uk/newsletter to sign up.

# Hope and Healing after Stillbirth and New Baby Loss

**Professor Kevin Gournay CBE** is a Chartered Psychologist, Registered Nurse and Chartered Scientist. He spent the first part of his career as a Registered Nurse working in various settings and then became one of the first professionals to receive training in cognitive behavioural therapy (then simply called behaviour therapy). Professor Gournay qualified as a psychologist having undertaken a range of research into the nature and treatment of anxiety disorders for his doctorate. He also received post-doctoral training in a number of health-related topics. Around 30 years ago Professor Gournay had the privilege of working in a palliative care service and, around the same time, had first-hand experience of stillbirth. Since then, Professor Gournay has seen a large number of women and their partners who have experienced stillbirth and perinatal death. He retired from his clinical work with patients in December 2018. He has also provided expert reports to courts, instructed by both solicitors acting for affected individuals and solicitors acting for the NHS. Professor Gournay has also acted as a patron and adviser to a number of charities in related areas.

Professor Gournay has research input to an initiative on drugs and alcohol and mental illness in Australia. He lives in Hertfordshire with his family and has four children. In his spare time, he enjoys running and has been a supporter of Charlton Athletic Football Club for over 50 years.

**Dr Brenda Ashcroft** qualified as a midwife in 1974. She worked for a few years as a hospital midwife, gaining experience in all areas. She spent many years working as a Community Midwifery Sister, providing care in a variety of settings, including the home, GP surgeries and health centres. During this time, she also undertook home deliveries and births in a GP unit similar to the birth centres in use today. She undertook an Advanced Diploma in Midwifery in 1988 and a teaching qualification in 1989. After this she worked as a Midwifery Tutor and then Midwifery Lecturer at the University of Salford. She obtained an MA in Health Care Ethics and Law in 1996 and a PhD in 2006. Her PhD research involved identifying risk in seven labour wards in the North West of England and the underlying causes of 37 cases of severe birth asphyxia with a potential to result in cerebral palsy. All cases involved negligence. She has contributed to the work of Sands and the King's Report on Safe Births, and presented her work to government organizations and on television and radio.

Since formally retiring at the end of July 2011, she provides occasional lectures to midwives and neonatal nurses at the University of Salford. In the last few years she has worked as an expert witness in many legal cases involving stillbirth, perinatal death and cerebral palsy.